COMMUNICATION AND LANGUAGE INTERVENTION PROGRAM (CLIP)

COMMUNICATION AND LANGUAGE INTERVENTION PROGRAM (CLIP)

for Individuals with Moderate to Severe Handicaps

By

JANE Y. MURDOCK, Ph.D.

Associate Professor
Department of Special Education
University of New Orleans
New Orleans, Louisiana

and

BARBARA V. HARTMANN, M.A.

Director, Speech-Language-Hearing Clinic
Assistant Clinical Professor
Speech-Language Pathology and Audiology
University of Utah
Salt Lake City, Utah

THOMAS BOOKS · SYMBOL OF LEADERSHIP

CHARLES C THOMAS • PUBLISHER
Springfield • Illinois • U.S.A.

Published and Distributed Throughout the World by

CHARLES C THOMAS • PUBLISHER
2600 South First Street
Springfield, Illinois 62717

ISBN 0-398-05095-3

Library of Congress Catalog Card Number: 84-23997

With THOMAS BOOKS *careful attention is given to all details of manufacturing and design. It is the Publisher's desire to present books that are satisfactory as to their physical qualities and artistic possibilities and appropriate for their particular use.* THOMAS BOOKS *will be true to those laws of quality that assure a good name and good will.*

Printed in the United States of America
Q-R-3

Library of Congress Cataloging in Publication Data

Murdock, Jane Y.
Communication and language intervention program (CLIP) for Individuals with Moderate to Severe Handicaps

Includes bibliographical references and index.
1. Communicative disorders — Treatment. 2. Speech therapy. I. Hartmann, Barbara V. II. Title.
RC423.M74 1985 616.85'52 84-23997
ISBN 0-398-05095-3

To Merlin J. Mecham

CONTENTS

COMMUNICATION AND LANGUAGE INTERVENTION PROGRAM (CLIP)

CHAPTER 1

PHILOSOPHY AND OVERVIEW

JANE Y. MURDOCK

THE ability to use language is the uniquely human trait, more so than standing upright or having an opposing thumb and fingers. Communicating about things present and not present and things dreamed about is the characteristic that sets Homo sapiens apart from other animals. Tragically, there are many inividuals who stand upright, have opposing thumb and fingers and all of the other human characteristics, but they are lacking the uniquely human characteristic. They do not use language. Missing the distinctive trait places a burden on noncommunicative humans that few of us can fathom. Providing that trait allows them to step over the threshold, welcomed by other communicating humans. This *Communication and Language Intervention Program* (CLIP) is an attempt to make that step possible.

The terms *communication* and *language* are often used interchangeably. However, they are not synonymous terms and some distinction between the two is necessary. Communication is the broader term and includes language. Communication involves any sharing of information between at least two participants, one who is the sender and the other who is the receiver. Furthermore, to qualify as communication, it must have some effect on the receiver. Eye contact is a form of communication. Smiling, frowning, waving, shaking hands, and body posture and positioning are all forms of communication.

Language is also a form of communication. However, any given language community develops much more complex rules to govern its usage than apply to other forms of communication. These rules can be semantic (rule for meaning), pragmatic (rules for meaning in context), phonological (rules for combining sounds), syntactic (rules for word order and structure), and morphological (rules for word form and structure). While language is usually spoken or written, it can also be signed or involve sequencing a variety of symbols that vary in their level of abstraction. Throughout this text the emphasis will be on teaching moderately to severely communicatively impaired individuals to communicate within the context of their natural environments, using whatever forms of communication that are available to them.

PHILOSOPHY

This is a behavioral approach to communication and language instruction. Consequently, our primary concern is not with what caused the disability but rather with identifying an individual's strengths and weaknesses, as well as his or her total communication and language needs. However, many of those who will benefit from this approach are typically labeled autistic, childhood or developmentally aphasic, severe language/learning disabled, or moderately to severely mentally retarded. Very often the person who is severely communicatively impaired has multiple handicaps, frequently including, but not limited to, some combination of the above, along with cerebral palsy or other motor disabilities which physically limit the ability to communicate successfully. Consequently, the program's focus is not only on spoken receptive and expressive language but on other aspects of communication that can enhance the possibility of learning to communicate successfully.

Whenever possible, teach communicative tasks in natural environments in the home, school, and community. When this is not possible because of restrictive regulations or practical considerations that prevent your working in the home or the community, make a concerted effort to involve teachers, parents, and others in the instructional process and teach communicative skills related to real objects in the natural environments that you do have access to and to real or simulated objects and actions in the classroom or clinic. If none of the above arrangements can be accommodated, photographs, pictures, and other substitutes can be used.

There are instances where it is desirable to gradually shift teaching materials from real objects in natural environments to materials that are commonly used and readily accessible in typical classrooms. With the present mandate to provide educational services in least restrictive environments, it is becoming more and more possible for the moderately to severely handicapped student to move from residential institutions, self-contained schools, or self-contained classrooms into integrated educational settings. Therefore, many speech pathologists and other special educators take the position that it is their responsibility to prepare their students for a successful transition by gradually shifting to materials that are at least similar to those that they will encounter in the typical classroom environment.

Who Can Use This Program?

CLIP is designed as a guide for speech-language pathologists, special educators, regular classroom teachers, psychologists, parents, and paraprofessionals who are working with individuals who have moderate to severe communication and language disorders. These disorders may vary considerably. In their most severe forms the child, adolescent, or adult may be totally nonverbal. She does not talk, she does not appear to understand what she hears or sees, and she does not respond to communicative gestures and postures. Milder manifestations include an individual who may understand most of what he hears and sees, that is, he has excellent receptive communication and language skills and he may have some speech. However, he has not mastered the spoken grammar that is typical of a normal child who is 3½ or 4 years old.

OVERVIEW

How to Assess Communication and Language Behaviors

Begin by taking the spontaneous communication and language samples described in Chapter 2. These are part of your preprogram observations. It is essential to discover how the individual is presently communicating, whether she is speaking, signing, using a symbol system such as Bliss symbols, gesturing, or failing to communicate. The spontaneous communication and language samples provide information regarding eye contact, body language, vocalizations, touching, stress and rhythm patterns, intonation, as well as morphological and syntactic structures the student understands or generates. These samples are taken at least two or three times in each of three different settings — ideally school, home, and community.

Guidelines Regarding What to Teach

Moderately to severely communicatively impaired students must constantly expand their receptive and expressive vocabularies. However, functional communication goes much further. It involves learning to: (1) follow instructions, (2) make requests, (3) interact socially with greetings or other polite communications, (4) describe things, (5) reject things, (6) comment on others' communications, activities, objects, etc., (7) and use communication and language forms to control self and others. Procedures for obtaining spontaneous communication and language samples in order to determine precisely what communicative skills an individual student needs to learn are described in Chapter 2. Table 2-1 provides a format for recording general communicative behaviors, as well as antecedent and consequent environmental events related to such behaviors. Table 2-2 provides a checklist of general communicative efforts. Table

2-3 provides developmentally based guidelines for analyzing syntactic and morphological structures. The data recorded on these three tables provide an overall picture of current and needed communication and receptive and expressive language skills within natural environments.

The spontaneous language samples also provide information regarding *body language* and *paralanguage.* Body language includes eye contact, facial expressions, body posture, and head and body orientation, as well as the obvious communicative hand gestures. Paralanguage involves the ability to respond to and use effective intonation and rhythm patterns, including pitch, stress, pauses, and vocal inflections. According to Bzoch and League (1971), these are among the earliest communicative acts. While it is generally accepted that most communication is accomplished verbally, paralanguage and body language are also critical to effective communication (Higginbotham & Yoder, 1982). Mehrabian (1972) suggests that only 7 percent of the total communication is carried by the actual choice of words, while 38 percent is carried by paralanguage and the remaining 55 percent by body language.

Chapter 3 contains descriptions of communicative behaviors that should be reinforced (taught), beginning with eye contact and ending with receptive and expressive language. Samples of morphological and syntactic structures normally used by children who are 3½ to 4 years old are provided in Table 3-1. These samples provide models which you can use to plug in the morphology and syntax that are relevant to use with a particular individual.

An "Ordered List of Environmentally Useful Words" assembled by one of the authors of this program is included in Appendix A (cf. Hartmann, 1975). Language instructors may use this list to help them select words that are appropriate for each individual. The words are listed from those that are easier to those that are more difficult to pronounce. Actual objects and/or pictures of the words in the "Ordered List of Environmentally Useful Words" are usually available in most home, school, and/or community settings.

How to Teach Communication and Language Behaviors

General instructions are presented in Chapter 2. Detailed teaching procedures are presented in Chapter 3, beginning with an emphasis on teaching in natural environments and ending with how to establish attending and eliminate interfering behaviors. The following presents a brief description of intervention procedures covered in Chapter 3.

How to Establish Communication and Language Behaviors

You must determine what antecedent or *discriminative stimuli* you will present. Put very simply, discriminative stimuli include all the things you say and do *before* an anticipated response from the individual you are instructing in order to get the response you desire. Specific structures, examples of those structures, and possible questions designed to evoke those structures are described in detail in Table 3-1 and Table 3-2 presents a sample teaching format for syntactic and morphological structures that corresponds with Table 3-1. This teaching format includes visual and auditory discriminative stimuli, prompting procedures, criteria for correct responding, and consequent stimuli. Additional information is included in Chapter 3 regarding tactile and kinesthetic stimuli that may be necessary in order to evoke desired communicative responses from severely handicapped individuals. These particularly relate to teaching appropriate stress and rhythm patterns and body language.

Typically, discriminative stimuli involve instructuring or telling an individual what you want him to do within a particular context. If simple instructions fail, model or otherwise prompt the student to respond correctly. If instructing, modeling, or prompting are unsuccessful, it may be necessary to shape the communicative behavior you desire. Detailed instructing, modeling, prompting, and shaping procedures are provided in Chapter 3.

How to Maintain and Strengthen Communication and Language Behaviors

Reinforce desirable communicative behaviors in order to maintain or strengthen them. The principles of reinforcement are very simple. You present something that is positive or remove something that is aversive immediately following any response you wish to maintain or strengthen. The crux of the matter, however, is determining *what* is positive or aversive for any given person. You will learn a great deal about what is reinforcing for each individual you plan to instruct while taking the spontaneous communication and language samples described in Chapter 2. Chapter 2 also contains detailed information about how to select reinforcers. The cardinal rule is: *Never assume without empirical data that you know what will reinforce (strengthen the behavior of) another living thing.*

Responsive Teaching and Accountability

Recording and Graphing Data

Procedures for recording and graphing data are described in Chapter 4. These procedures are simplified so that they will provide feedback for instructors about the effectiveness of their instruction. Instructors who are responsive to these data will not only teach more effectively but, as a consequence of having more successful teaching experiences, should find teaching itself more rewarding (Hall, 1971; Hall, 1974).

Figure 4-1 is a sample data recording sheet which is coordinated with Table 3-2, the sample teaching format. These simplify lesson planning and record keeping. All immediately relevant information for a student or a group of students can be marked quickly on the data recording sheet. Space is provided that corresponds to the directions on the sample teaching format. The communication and language instructor simply fills in each section of the data recording sheet with a brief description of the communication and language tasks. She will then have before her a single sheet which provides information regarding precisely what is to be taught, what kind of reinforcers to present, the reinforcement schedule for each particular communicative task, the prompting procedures for each task, exactly what to say and do to evoke correct responding, and space to record the data.

Keeping accurate data is essential to the success of this program. Furthermore, data have to be presented in a form that is easy to repond to and interpret. This can be accomplished by using the data recording and graphing procedures described in Chapter 4.

Single-Subject Research Designs

While simply recording and graphing data provide some evidence about what an individual is learning, they do not provide any evidence regarding *why* the learning is occurring or if, in fact, your teaching is responsible. Fortunately, there are several research designs that can be used by teachers, parents, and others that will demonstrate a cause-effect relationship between instructional procedures (independent variables) and what the instructed individuals learned (dependent variables). These are in Chapter 4 and include an AB design, a reversal design, a multiple baseline design, a changing criterion design, an alternating treatments design, and a changing conditions design (Alberto & Troutman, 1982; Baer, Wolf, & Risley, 1968; Hall, 1974; Hartmann & Hall, 1976; Hersen & Barlow, 1976; Sidman, 1960).

These designs provide for systematic replication of your communication and language intervention strategies. They demonstrate that you are responsible for the learning that has occurred; that you are accountable for your instructional decisions. Accountability requirements have become some of the most time-consuming responsibilities of speech pathologists and educators. Following the procedures set forth in Chapter 4 will clearly demonstrate your accountability. Indeed, following these procedures may prove to be the biggest boon for you as the communication and language instructor, because you will know that any progress made was not some fortuitous accident but was a direct result of your efforts.

Planning in Advance for Generalization

Chapter 5 provides guidelines to ensure that, once mastered, communication and language behaviors will generalize appropriately (Murdock, Garcia, & Hardman, 1977; Stokes & Baer, 1977). By arranging for instruction in natural environments and providing more than one instructor from the outset, you have greatly enhanced the likelihood that the individual will use and generalize what she has learned. To ascertain whether acquired behaviors are generalizing appropriately, use the generalization probing and training procedures described in Chapter 5. The ultimate test of communicative competence is how persistent the behaviors are and whether or not a person can communicate appropriately: (1) in other physical settings where no specific teaching has occurred, (2) with other people who have never participated in any training, (3) when presented with different instructions or other antecedent stimuli, such as different objects or events, and (4) with different but similar communicative acts. This latter often implies that some basic rule-governed language behaviors have become internalized. If your probing procedures reveal that appropriate generalization has not occurred, specific generalization training procedures are provided in Chapter 5.

How to Deliver Communication and Language Services

A service delivery model is described in Chapter 6. For the majority of severely communicatively handicapped individuals, teaching language and communication skills is more successful if they are taught continuously throughout their waking hours and in natural environments where those skills are needed. There is good evidence that communication and language skills are acquired more readily within such natural contexts (Bates, 1979; Bruner, 1975; MacDonald & Hortsmeier, 1978; McLean & Snyder-McLean, 1978).

Furthermore, one of the most pervasive problems we have with moderately to severely communicatively impaired individuals is their failure to generalize behaviors that have been acquired in contrived learning environments such as those that prevail in most school or clinics (Brookshire, 1967; Engel, Brandriet, Erickson, Gronhovd, & Gunderson, 1966; Johnston & Johnston, 1972; Kazdin & Bootzin, 1972; Mulac & Tomlinson, 1977; Murdock, Garcia, & Hardman, 1977; Schuler, 1980). This is true of both stimulus generalization (the ability to demonstrate acquired behaviors in settings other than those where training occurred) and response generalization (responding with new behaviors which are similar to those specifically trained). There is evidence that much of the generalization dilemma can be alleviated if people are taught in their natural environments, in situations where they actually need to use the communicative forms and can receive naturally occurring consequences for their communicative attempts (Carr, 1980; Carr & Kologinsky, 1983; Cavallaro, 1983; Hart & Risley, 1974; Hart & Risley, 1975; Hart & Risley, 1980; Hart & Rogers-Warren, 1978; Koegel & Rincover, 1974; Kopchick & Lloyd, 1976; McGee, Krantz, Mason, & McClannahan, 1983; Nietupski, Scheutz, & Ockwood, 1980; Rogers-Warren & Warren, 1980; Schuler, 1980). In order to enhance both acquisition and generalization, milieu and incidental teaching models are reviewed in Chapter 6. Chapter 6 concludes with CLIP's service delivery model.

Implications for Reaching More Communicatively Impaired Individuals

As a result of this service delivery model, many more moderately to severely communicatively impaired individuals can receive the communication and language instruction they need and are legally entitled to receive. However, the role of the highly trained specialist will become one of not only delivering direct services but also of providing on-site training about how to teach communication and language for teachers, paraprofessionals, parents, and others. In our experience, this model provides for more effective in-service training than meeting with teachers, paraprofessionals, parents, etc., once a week on Friday afternoon (or less) and hoping they will apply what you have told them next Monday or whenever they next interact with the individuals with whom we are concerned.

What About Individuals Who Cannot Talk?

While much of the emphasis of this program is on teaching moderately to severely communicatively impaired individuals to understand and use spoken language, there are several alternative forms of communication available which are covered in Chapter 7. The major objective is to teach individuals with severe communication disorders to communicate by the most effective way or ways available to them (Carr, 1980; Carr & Kologinsky, 1983; Murdock, 1978b; Schaeffer, 1980; Schaeffer, Musil, & Kollinzas, 1980; Scheifelbusch, 1980). Speaking is only one form of communication, although granted it is highly desirable because it is the most readily understood. However, placing the individual's needs first, we feel that it is essential to provide any viable form of expressive communication that is available. The particular form is secondary. Many people for a variety of known and unknown reasons do not learn to speak, but they can learn to use gestures, signing, symbol systems, or augmentative language devices to express themselves. In some instances this seems to provide them with the vehicle to use spoken language (Schaeffer, 1980). The better known symbol system modes, visual-motor communication systems, combined modes, and augmentative communication techniques are discussed in Chapter 7.

The teaching procedures in CLIP are as relevant for teaching manual communication or other communication forms as they are for teaching spoken language. Whether you are teaching symbol systems, signing, speaking, or some combination of these, this program will provide guidelines about what to teach, as well as how, when, and where to teach it.

Applications of Computer Techology

Prosthetic devices that can provide speech for the nonspeaking are, perhaps, the most impressive contributions that computer technology has made for moderately to severely communicatively impaired individuals. Many of these are reviewed in Chapter 8. In addition, computer-managed instruction (CMI) and computer-assisted instruction (CAI) are reviewed. Chapter 8 also includes an example of an easy-to-develop software program and concludes with the creative potential for using computer technology to teach moderately to severely communicatively impaired individuals.

CHAPTER 2

PREPROGRAM OBSERVATIONS AND GENERAL INSTRUCTIONS

JANE Y. MURDOCK and BARBARA V. HARTMANN

THIS chapter specifies the overall objectives of CLIP and procedures for taking spontaneous communication and language samples during preprogram observations. General instructions about how to reinforce or strengthen behaviors, how to select reinforcers, and the importance of using a multisensory approach to teaching communication and language skills are also provided. Read these general instructions thoroughly before attempting to use the communication and language placement and intervention procedures described in CLIP.

OBJECTIVES

A communicatively impaired person who successfully completes this entire communication and language intervention plan will be able to do the following:

1. Understand and use environmentally useful vocabulary, including that which is relevant from Appendix A.
2. Follow instructions.
3. Communicate intelligibly. This does not imply speaking with perfect articulation but rather with understandable speech, signs, symbols, or augmented communication.
4. Make requests.
5. Interact socially with greetings and other polite communications.
6. Describe things.
7. Reject things.

8. Comment on objects, activities, and comments made by others.
9. Use communicative skills to control behavior of self and others.
10. Communicate with eye contact, facial expressions, gestures, and body posture and positioning.
11. Communicate with effective rhythm, inflection, and intonation patterns.
12. Use appropriate morphological forms and syntactic structures in five- to seven-word sentences.
13. Generalize communication and language mastered in instructional environments to: (1) settings where no specific instruction occurred, (2) people who did not participate specifically in communication or language instruction, (3) different discriminative stimuli, and (4) similar communication and language tasks.

PREPROGRAM OBSERVATIONS

Before beginning instruction, videotape or tape record spontaneous communication and language samples for at least two 10-minute periods in at least three major environments: (1) areas related to teaching/learning, such as school, (2) areas related to home and/or home living skills, such as the actual home or simulated home environments in the school or institution, and (3) areas related to the community, such as grocery stores, restaurants, playgrounds, laundromats, or bowling alleys. These major environments are not mutually exclusive but may overlap considerably. It is also noteworthy that both work and recreational activities occur in all of them. Ideally, these observations should be videotaped. However, for verbal students, tape recording may be sufficient. We encourage the videotaping because accurate observations of the student's total communication attempts can be made. Tape recordings cannot be used with nonspeaking students. Furthermore, they provide only the auditory component of the communication of those who do speak. Videotaped samples can be used to a far greater extent than tape recordings to complete the spontaneous communication and language sample records in Table 2-1, the checklist in Table 2-2, and the record of syntactic and morphological structures in Table 2-3. You will have a minimum of 60 minutes of spontaneous communication and language samples.

If you cannot obtain spontaneous communication and language samples in the recommended environments as desired above, select a variety of settings that are available to you for this purpose. Ideally, one of these settings should be a highly structured setting, such as a matching-like-objects session; one fairly unstructured activity, such as storytime; and one totally unstructured setting, such as freetime at school. If at all possible, get similar samples at home as well. If traveling to the student's home is not feasible, invite the parents or others in the home environment to come to the school so that you can observe and, ideally, videotape their interactions.

TABLE 2-1

EXAMPLES OF SPONTANEOUS COMMUNICATION AND LANGUGE SAMPLE RECORDS

	Student's Response		
Setting Place, Objects, People, And/or On-going Activity	Probable Communicative Intent	Communicative Attempt	Consequent Events After Student Responds
Example 1			
Cottage of large residential school.	Wants to use the toilet	Looks at teacher	Teacher looks at student.
Teacher, aid, six severely retarded adolescents.	Wants to use the toilet	Looks and points sort of in the direction of the bathroom.	Teacher looks and asks. "What do you want?"
	Wants to use the toilet	Looks and points in the direction of the bathroom and tugs at her jeans.	Teacher looks and says, "Oh, you want to go to the bathroom! Good telling me. Let's go!"
Example 2			
Classroom. Blocks.	Wants big block	Points	No response
Two peers.	Wants big block	Points, grunts	No response
	Wants big block	Points, grunts, pushes pile of blocks down	Peer looks, says "No!"
	Wants big block	Grabs block	Peer hits him
Example 3			
Grocery store.	Wants to pay the clerk	Stands at check out	Clerk looks at her
Teacher, clerk, four customers in line behind student.	Wants to pay the clerk	Stands at checkout	Clerk looks at her and holds out hand for money.
	Wants to pay the clerk	Stands at checkout and looks at her teacher	Teacher looks at and touches student's purse
Example 4			
School hallway. Mother and child.	Doesn't want to go home	"Tay"	No response
Mother putting on child's coat	Doesn't want to go home	"Tay here."	No response
	Doesn't want to go home	"Me tay here."	"No, we have to go home!" Jerks child's arm.
	Doesn't want to go home	"Please, me tay here."	"I'm sorry. We have to go home and see Bobby now." Hugs child.

Table 2-1 (Continued)

Example 5

Integrated high school Retarded 16-yr-old male, and teacher. Verbal outburst of student following psychological testing.	Wants to apologize for making a scene	Sideward glance with no direct eye contact	Looks at student
	Wants to apologize for making a scene	Direct eye contact followed by dropping head slightly.	Looks at student and nods head slightly as though disappointed.
	Wants to apologize for making a scene	Raises head and says, "Okay, I'm sorry I shot my mouth off, but I've taken those (pause) *tests* a hundred times!"	Slaps student gently on the shoulder and says, "It's part of what we've got go do to get you into a classroom. I'm calling Dr. Blank back here now and I'm counting on you to hang in. There's not that much left to do!"

Spontaneous Communication and Language Samples

General Observations. Use the sixty minutes of recorded observations to explore the communication and language requirements of the student in school, at home, in the community generally, and in areas where he will play or enjoy other forms of recreation. See Table 2-1 for examples of how to record spontaneous communication and language samples.

Use spontaneous communication and language sample records to record: (1) the setting, (2) the communicative intent, (3) the communicative attempt, and (4) the consequent events. The entire spontaneous communication and language sample record can be written descriptively or the following codes can be used. These codes are particularly useful when you have to rely on tape recordings since you will have to make notations about nonauditory stimuli as they occur.

NR = No response
EC- = No eye contact
EC+ = Eye contact
BL+ = Positive body language
BL- = Punitive body language
G = Communicative gestures
VN = Nonintentional vocalization
V+ = Intentional positive vocalization
V- = Intentional punitive vocalization
VV+ = Successful vocal verbalization
VV- = Unsuccessful vocal verbalization
T+ = Communicative touching
T- = Noncommunicative touching

SR+ = Appropriate stress and rhythm patterns
SR- = Inappropriate stress and rhythm patterns
P+ = Appropropriate pauses
P- = Inappropriate pauses
I+ = Normal intonation
I- = Abnormal intonation

Check each of the communicative behaviors in Table 2-2. Simple yes/no responses are required for items 1 through 21. More detailed written responses are required for items 22 through 27.

TABLE 2-2

SPONTANEOUS COMMUNICATION AND LANGUAGE SAMPLE CHECKLIST

	Yes	No
1. Does the student respond to his own name? (V)	_____	_____
2. Does the student make or respond to eye contact? (EC)	_____	_____
3. Does he reach for objects or persons, initiating such an action or in response to objects or persons being presented to him? (G)	_____	_____
4. Does he orient his head or body in response to communicative gestures? (V & BL)	_____	_____
5. Does he whine or cry to communicate his needs or desires? (V)	_____	_____
6. Does he use vocalizations that approximate normal rhythm patterns? (V)	_____	_____
7. Are vocalizations accompanied with communicative gestures? (V & BL)	_____	_____
8. Does he touch others to gain their attention? (BL & G)	_____	_____
9. Does he repeat what others say, using exactly the same tone of voice, inflections, etc. (immediate echolalia)?	_____	_____
10. Does he use social language forms such as "Hi" or "Bye-bye?" (V)	_____	_____
11. Does he attempt to communicate his desires?	_____	_____
12. Does he attempt to control the behavior of others?	_____	_____
13. Does he describe things?	_____	_____
14. Does he reject things?	_____	_____
15. Does he take turns?	_____	_____
16. Does he share?	_____	_____
17. Does he refer to objects and/or things not immediately present?	_____	_____
18. Does he express personal feelings?	_____	_____
19. Does he try to inform people about things he would assume they know nothing about?	_____	_____
20. Does he ask questions?	_____	_____
21. Do people respond positively to his communicative efforts?	_____	_____

22. How does he communicate now (e.g., speech, Bliss symbols, communication board, manual communication, etc.)?
23. How do people gain his attention?
24. How do people respond to his communicative attempts? Do they ignore him? Punish him? Reward him?
25. What rewards do people give him that are the most effective?
26. What communicative forms, including words, gestures, signs, symbols, etc., does he need to be able to use immediately?
27. What grammatical constructions are people using that he does not appear to understand?

SPECIFIC OBSERVATIONS. Use these videotaped or tape-recorded communication and language samples to complete as much as possible of the morphological and syntactic structures in Table 2-3. You may get most of the information that you need about the student's communication skills by carefully analyzing these preprogram recordings, in which case it would not be necessary to directly administer the items in Table 2-3.

TABLE 2-3

SYNTACTIC AND MORPHOLOGICAL STRUCTURES

A. A student's syntax and morphology are readily available for evaluation from the videotapes or recordings you made in your preprogram observations. Take the spontaneous communication and language samples which you recorded and compare them to the "Correct Responses" described in "Column 1." Indicate whether the student spontaneously used these by writing the responses in or by marking a plus (+) or a minus (-) under the description of the correct response. Note whether the communication is spoken, written, signed, or some other symbol system. For responses in "Column 1" that a student failed to make spontaneously, follow the procedures in B through D below.

B. Normally, it is not necessary to test in any stage that is prior to and, consequently, less difficult than a stage in which the student *did* succeed. For example, if a student said, "My shoes are wet," when indeed they were wet and he was not just immediately imitating or making a nonfunctional echolalic utterance, he has made an appropriate response for stage D. Therefore, do not require him to say phrases that are grammatically acceptable for a developing student but which are not grammatically acceptable for an adult, e.g., "Throw ball box," in stage C.

C. In instances where you did *not* get a spontaneous language sample in the natural environment which was at or above the stage you are testing in, present the following:
   1. Perform each action in "Column 2" and record the student's spontaneous responses in the space provided below the description of your action.
   2. If the above fails to evoke the desired response spontaneously, ask each question in "Column 3" and record the student's responses in the space provided below your question.
   3. If the student has not yet given the response you are testing, model it for him as described in "Column 4" and record the student's imitation in the space provided below the description of your model.

D. Discontinue testing in any stage when the student makes three errors in response to your model in "Column 4."

E. Begin teaching in any stage where it was necessary to model the correct response. It is not necessary to teach in a stage where the student responded correctly to the situation or to appropriate questions for all items in that stage."

Stage A

COLUMN 1	COLUMN 2	COLUMN 3	COLUMN 4
Record of spontaneous language sample taken during preprogram observations.	Action — May repeat once	Question — May repeat once	Model — May repeat twice

---

The format for Table 2-3 is adapted from *Environmental Language Inventory* (MacDonald & Nickols, 1974).

Table 2-3 (Continued)

Correct response:			
Two or more words that include the name of an object.	Make a toy appear suddenly.	"What do you say?"	"Say, 'Hi, (Gilbert).'" "Say, 'That's a (doll).'"
Two or more words that indicate a request for "more."	Give student a small toy or bit of edible.	"What do you want?"	"Say, 'More banana.'" "Say, 'Another bite.'" (Student may say "'nother.'")
Two or more words that indicate the ability to ask or talk about something that cannot be seen.	Show toy. Cover with blanket.	"What do you say?"	"Say, 'Where's (Gil)?'" "Say, '(Gilbert) gone.'" "Say, 'No (Gilbert).'"

Stage B

COLUMN 1	COLUMN 2	COLUMN 3	COLUMN 4
Record of spontaneous language sample taken during preprogram observations.	Action — May repeat once	Question — May repeat once	Model — May repeat twice
Correct response:			
Two or more words that express acting on an object.	Perform action with toy.	"What did I do?" "What do you want to do?"	"Say, 'Throw the (ball).'" "Say, 'Push the (car).'" (Student may omit *the*.)
Two or more words that express a subject performing an action.	Doll or toy animal does action (with no object).	"What's going on?"	"Say, 'Baby's crying.'" "Say, 'Puppy's sleeping." (Student may omit *'s* & *-ing*.)
One word "mine" is acceptable here, as well as any two or more words that express the student's possession.	In fun, take something belonging to student.	"Whose is this?"	"Say, 'My (ball).'"
Two or more words that express location of one object in relation to another. The actual preposition is not required here.	Put toy on a chair, table, etc.	"Where's the (car)?" "How about the (baby)?"	"Say, 'Car's on the chair.'" "Say, 'Baby's on the table.'" (Student my omit *'s*, and *the*.)

Table 2-3 (Continued)

Two or more words that express the size relationship of one object to the other.	Show two objects out of reach, one noticeably big, the other little.	"Which do you want?"	"Say, 'Big (block).'" "Say, 'Little (block).'"
Stage C — Word Order			
COLUMN 1 Record of spontaneous language sample taken during preprogram observations.	COLUMN 2 Action — May repeat once	COLUMN3 Question — May repeat once	COLUMN 4 Model — May repeat twice
Correct Response:			
Three or more words that indicate a subject acting on an object.	Doll or toy animal does something with an object.	"What Happened?"	"Say, 'Baby threw the ball.'" "Say, 'Puppy ate the cookie.'" (Student may omit *the*.)
Three or more words that indicate an action and the relationship between two objects.	Offer two destinations or containers and begin to throw or push object(s).	"What should I do?"	"Say, 'Throw the ball in the box.'" "Say, 'Push the car to the door.'" (Student may omit *the, in, to*)
Three or more words that indicate wanting something that varies in size.	Offer big and little blocks, Tinkertoys®, etc., repeatedly.	"What do you say?"	"Say, 'More big blocks.'" "Say, 'Another little stick.'" (Student may say, "'Nother")
Three or more words that include the word "no" to indicate the opposite action.	Doll, toy animal, or student does something.	Describe the opposite action.	"Say, 'Puppy does not jump!'" "Say, 'I do not hide.'" (Student may omit *does* & *do*)
Three or more words that ask a "what" plus subject and verb.	Perform action with object where student can't see.	"I'm eating something. "I just made someting.	"Say, 'What are you eating?'" "Say, 'What did you make?'" (Student may omit *are, did, -ing*)
Stage C — Word Form			
COLUMN 1 Record of spontaneous language sample taken during preprogram observations.	COLUMN 2 Action — May repeat once	COLUMN 3 Question — May repeat once	COLUMN 4 Model — May repeat twice

Table 2-3 (Continued)

Two or more words that include verb plus -ing.	Doll, tester or toy does a continuous action.	"What's happening?"	"Say, 'It's sleeping.'" "Say, 'You're eating.'" (Student may omit *'s* and *'re*)
One plural response	Offer one desired object and then two or more of the same object.	"What do you want?"	"Say, 'Marble*s*.'" "Say, 'Block*s*.'"
Two to four words that include I, me, my (and) a, an, and the.	Look at previously recorded spontaneous utterances for: I, me, my (and) a, an, and the.		"Say, '*I* want a ball.'" "Say, 'Give *me the* ball.'" "Say, 'It's *my* baby.'" "Say, 'Give me *an* apple.'"

Testing Instructions for Stages D through F

1. Analyze the videotapes or other recordings of the student's spontaneous language. Select the longer spontaneous examples of the following syntactic or morphological forms and record them in "Column 1." For those not found, use the procedures in 2 through 5.
2. Based upon the average length of the spontaneous language sample utterances, choose to model *either* the three- to four- or the five- to seven-word sentences listed below.
3. Model the sentences in either "Column 2" or "Column 3," asking the student to say what you say. The structures to be tested are in italics in each sentence.
4. Each model may be repeated once if necessary, but return to it after another sentence has been presented.
5. Record the student's response in the space provided directly below the sentence he is attempting to imitate.

Stage D — Word Order

COLUMN 1	COLUMN 2	COLUMN 3
Spontaneous Language	3-4 Word Sentences	5-6 Word Sentences
's contraction	"Mom'*s* mad."	"My dad'*s* very big."
is plus verb*ing*	"Daddy *is* sleeping."	"My mommy *is* sleeping upstairs."
'll	"I'*ll* do it."	"I'*ll* pour my own milk."
will	"I *will* go."	"I *will* pour my milk."

Stage D — Word Form

COLUMN 1	COLUMN 2	COLUMN 3
Spontaneous Language Sample	3-4 Word Sentences	5-6 Word Sentences
+*s* possessive	"It's Mom'*s* coat."	"It's my Mom'*s* coat."
they	"*They* want candy."	"*They* watch TV every night."

Stage E — Word Order

are	"My shoes *are* wet."	"Now my shoes *are* wet."
are + verb*ing*	"The dogs *are* barking."	"The dogs *are* barking outside."
Do question	"*Do* you live here?"	"*Do* you live in this house?"

Table 2-3 (Continued)

Stage E — Word Form

COLUMN 1	COLUMN 2	COLUMN 3
Spontaneous Language Sample	3-4 Word Sentences	5-7 Word Sentences
she + *s* action word	"*She* like*s* donuts."	"*She* like*s* donuts and milk."
we + *ed*	"*We* wash*ed* the car."	"*We* wash*ed* the car last Saturday."
	Stage F — Word Form and Word Order	
were + action*ing*	"The dogs *were* barking."	"The dogs *were* barking last night."
was + action*ing*	"Daddy *was* sleeping."	"Daddy *was* sleepig on the sofa."
because, so, etc.	"*Because* I'm tired."	"I'll go *because* I'm tired."
Wh question + *are*	"When *are* we going?"	"When *are* we going to Grandma's?

Making the above general and specific observations is necessary in order to: (1) complete the spontaneous communication language records in Table 2-1, the checklist in Table 2-2, and the sample morphological and syntactic structures in Table 2-3, (2) determine the communication, language, paralanguage, and body language skills which are immediately relevant and realistic for the student to learn, (3) list and evaluate the effectiveness of the student's current attempts to communicate, and (4) discover the consequences of his communicative attempts in his natural environment in order to select reinforcers that are already established that will fit into your particular teaching style. You will also discover environmental consequences that are punishing, thus weakening his communicative attempts. Furthermore, this is a good opportunity for you and the student to get to know each other.

Placement Procedures

Complete Tables 2-1, 2-2, and 2-3 to determine what communication and language skills to teach. Select spoken, written, signed, and other symbolic language skills; gestures and other body language skills; and paralanguage skills that the student can use immediately. Ideally, talk to both parents or guardians and teachers to supplement this list and the information you obtained during your preprogram observations.

In addition, take a survey of the community shops, restaurants, transportation, etc.; the recreational areas such as parks, movies, zoo, etc.; and present or future vocational sites. Combine all of these sources of information with the information you received from parents, teachers, and others and the records you kept during preprogram observations. These sources will result in meaningful content for communication and language instruction.

GENERAL INSTRUCTIONS

Reinforcing or Strengthening Behavior

When a behavior is reinforced, it becomes stronger or more likely to reoccur. Essentially, this is what teaching is about, strengthening desired behaviors. The principle of reinforcing behaviors in order to strengthen them is obvious (Alberto & Troutman, 1982; Axelrod, 1983; Bijou & Baer, 1967; Guess, Sailor & Baer, 1976; Hall, 1971; Hall, 1975; Murdock, 1978a; Murdock, Garcia, & Hardman, 1977; Murdock & Hartmann, 1975; Skinner, 1957; Sloane & MacAulay, 1968). However, determining what actually accomplishes this for each particular individual is not so obvious. We frequently make the mistake of assuming that something that we like is liked by everybody or that something that worked with Joey will also work with Maria. Such assumptions may be largely responsible for most teaching failures. In order to teach an individual to communicate, it is essential first to determine, and then to use, reinforcing consequences that will strengthen or increase the rate of his communicative behaviors.

Ultimately, communicative behaviors are reinforced as a result of naturally occurring consequences in the environment. This is one of the primary reasons why we have placed so much emphasis on teaching the communicatively impaired person in natural environments. If he is in the cafeteria and communicates that he wants a cookie and, consequently, receives a cookie, he is naturally reinforced for his communicative effort.

Unfortunately, with the moderately to severely communicatively impaired person, it frequently, at least initially, is necessary to use renforcers that are not necessarily natural to a particular situation. *Use whatever reinforcers you have to use to have a successful teaching/learning experience.* Once you establish the communicative behaviors, you can move away from contrived reinforcers and toward those that occur naturally.

Selecting Reinforcers

Much of the data needed for this section can be gathered during the preprogram observations. Your spontaneous communication and language sample records will provide information about how parents, teachers, and others interacting with the student reinforce her. Do they praise her? Touch her? Hug her? Give her tastes of banana or other edibles? Give her points or other tokens? Or provide some combination of the above? What seems to be the most effective? If they are keeping a record of the student's responses, look at their data to determine whether what they are doing is actually reinforcing the student. That is, is she learning what they are trying to teach her? Is the rate of appropriate communicative behaviors increasing or being strengthened? By definition, a reinforcer must strengthen the behavior that it follows unless that behavior is already at an optimal level, in which case a reinforcer maintains that level.

Given that all other instructional procedures and the level of the communicative skill you are attempting to teach are appropriate but, nevertheless, the student is not learning, an effective reinforcer has not been selected. When this situation exists, it will be necessary for you to offer her a variety of things that you think might be reinforcing while carefully keeping data in order to determine what the student chooses and whether the behaviors are strengthened. Data recording sheets similar to the example in Figure 4-1 can be used for this purpose. Although these are quite self-explanatory, you may wish to see Chapter 4 for detailed instructions about data recording procedures.

Also, keep a record of what the student does when she has a choice. Does she play with the record player? The blocks? The puzzles? Does she go outside to swing? Does she watch television? Play ball? Jump rope? Does she frequently approach a particular person? This information will give you a powerful reinforcer to use with her (Premack, 1959). These freely chosen objects or activities can be used as reinforcers by saying something like, "Okay, Denise, if you watch me, work hard, and listen today, we'll play on the swings (or whatever activity she prizes) when we're through," or "Tell me what we call these dishes and then you can help Ms. Andrews put the puzzle together." You can also use this information if the student is working on a point or token system because these items or activities can be used as backup reinforcers for her having earned a specified number of tokens.

You must continue to provide choices and vary what you offer to the student immediately after she responds correctly until the data you are recording indicate that communication and language behaviors are increasing or becoming stronger. In other words, she is learning. Keeping data is the only way you can know that you have found effective reinforcers.

One of the most important points to remember when trying to teach someone something is that each individual is unique. Therefore, consequences that increase or strengthen one person's behavior may not have the same effect for another person. This is as true for children as it is for adults. Some people will work very hard for praise or recognition. Others will only work very hard for tokens or money. Still others work very hard simply because they find something in the activity itself that is reinforcing.

Using a Multisensory Approach

Grace Fernald is probably the best known advocate of using multisensory stimulation when teaching handicapped learners (Myers & Hammill, 1976). The emphasis is upon involving visual, tactile, auditory and kinesthetic modalities in the instructional procedures (Fernald, 1943). Johnson and Myklebust (1964) recommend similar instructional procedures when they discuss the simultaneous pairing of language instruction with related experiences. However, for language instruction, Johnson and Myklebust particularly emphasize the auditory and visual modalities.

Regardless of the number of modalities involved, it is obvious that simply imitating spoken language or gestures is not an appropriate instructional procedure. Nevertheless, for many of us who are eager to teach the language handicapped individual gestures or words and how to string those words together so that she can communicate her needs, her desires, and her ideas, there is sometimes a tendency to forget that simply having her imitate a gesture or repeat the word after we say it is not enough. Teaching in natural environments automatically provides for multisensory stimulation and simultaneous pairing of relevant communication and language forms with the experiences they represent.

When circumstances do not permit teaching in natural environments, create a communication and language environment in which pairing the visual objects, activities, or pictures of objects or activities is integral. Otherwise, the student is simply learning to imitate gestures, sounds, words or sentences in a parrot-like fashion. Although *you* may know that these are communicative acts, for the student who is moderately to severely language impaired, they are not functioning as such unless she understands what they represent. This simultaneous pairing of the gesture or word with the things they represent will involve all of the relevant sensory stimuli, thus teaching her the meaning of the gestures or words you are teaching her to use as you are teaching her to use them (Johnson & Myklebust, 1964). This is critical to teaching *language* as opposed to teaching parrot-like, meaningless imitation of gestures, sounds, words and sentences. It is vitally important to teach communication and language skills while interacting with real objects that are important to her and in activities which occur often in her home, school, recreational, and community environments. The visual section of the sample teaching format in Chapter 3 is provided to make certain that this simultaneous pairing of at least the visual and auditory aspects of the communication is not inadvertently overlooked.

Simultaneously pairing the auditorily presented word with the visual or gestural representation of the word is just as critical for the person who is learning some form of visual expressive language, such as sign language, as it is for the person who is learning to speak. For both individuals, it is essential for you to pair the words with what they represent during communication and language training if they are to develop their *receptive* and *expressive* language by understanding what the word or the sign actually means. Often, hearing a word as it is visually represented by signs or symbols results in attempting to say the word as well (Schaeffer, 1980).

You are now ready to begin the teaching procedures described in Chapter 3.

CHAPTER 3

TEACHING PROCEDURES

JANE Y. MURDOCK and BARBARA V. HARTMANN

INSTRUCTIONAL SETTINGS

Individual and Group Instruction in Natural Environments

IN most instances, you will find that communication and language instruction can be conducted in environments where students need to use those particular communicative skills. For example, when you are teaching vocabulary and language structures related to food and eating, teach students at mealtime where the food, dishes, eating utensils, and other natural cues signal the desired communicative behaviors. Furthermore, naturally occurring consequences serve as reinforcers.

When you are teaching verbs, do so while students are engaging in, or watching others who are engaging in, the actions being taught. If you want them to learn about playground equipment or other vocabulary related to playground, do so when they would normally be in that environment or make special arrangements to take them to that environment (Carr, 1980; Cavallaro, 1983; Hart & Rogers-Warren, 1978; Schuler, 1980).

Teaching in natural environments helps to overcome one of the most pervasive problems we have with moderately to severely communicatively impaired individuals: They fail to generalize communicative behaviors that have been learned in contrived clinical or educational settings (Brookshire, 1967; Carr, 1980; Engel, Brandriet, Erickson, Gronhovd, & Gunderson, 1966; Johnston & Johnston, 1972; Kazdin & Bootzin, 1972; Mulac & Tomlinson, 1977, Schuler, 1980). For generalization purposes, it is also very important that you arrange to have others participate in language instruction (Cavallaro, 1983; Faw, Reid, Schepis, Fitzgerald, & Welty, 1981; Murdock, Garcia, & Hardman, 1977; Nietupski, Scheutz, & Ockwood, 1980; Stokes & Baer, 1977). When instruction occurs in natural environments, normally there will be several individuals who spontaneously become involved in teaching communication and language skills in very much the same manner that nonhandicapped children are taught. CLIP also provides procedures to train a wide variety of individuals to meet the special needs of moderately to severely communicatively impaired students, such as those described in the following section on language and communication instruction for individual students.

Individual Instruction in Temporarily Contrived Environments

With students who are new to the program or with severely multiply handicapped students, individual instruction may be necessary, at least initially. Provide this instruction by arranging an isolated area within the classroom, home, or other natural setting. This can be done simply by separating yourselves from the mainstream of ongoing activities, setting up screens or partitions if necessary.

Involve another adult instructor in the sessions from the beginning. This can be the classroom teacher, a parent, a paraprofessional, or a volunteer who comes in regularly. However, in an educational or clinical setting, the co-instructor should be someone who regularly interacts with or instructs two or three others in the same setting. For the first two or three sessions, the co-instructor will observe your instructional procedures, participating by sharing in delivering reinforcers. By the third or fourth session, the co-instructor will begin to share in the entire instructional process. Normally, the co-instructor will be able to assume the major instructional responsibility by the eighth session.

In the meantime, one, then two, and possibly even three or four of the co-instructor's other students are gradually introduced into the sessions. The screens or other barriers are also gradually removed until you are essentially instructing in a typical classroom environment.

The reasons for keeping the student within the mainstream as much as possible from the very beginning and for gradually phasing him into a totally natural setting are many; however, two are particularly important. One, there is good evidence that natural, contextual cues are important variables in the acquisition of communication skills (Bates, 1976; Bruner, 1975; MacDonald & Horstmeier, 1978; McLean & Snyder-McLean, 1978) and, two, delivering communication instruction in a natural environment greatly enhances the probability that the skills will generalize appropriately (Carr, 1980; Carr & Kologinsky, 1983; Cavallaro, 1983; Hart & Risley, 1974; Hart & Risley, 1975; Hart & Risley, 1980; Hart & Rogers-Warren, 1978; Koegel & Rincover, 1974; Kopchick & Lloyd, 1976; MacDonald & Horstmeier, 1978; McGee, Krantz, Mason, & McClannahan, 1983; McLean & Snyder-McLean, 1978; Nietupski, Scheutz, & Ockwood, 1980; Rogers-Warren & Warren, 1980; Schuler, 1980;

Stokes & Baer, 1977). Receiving instruction in natural environments will also help the student receive considerably more communication and language instruction than he could from a single speech pathologist. Furthermore, these procedures help to ensure that he will be able to learn from more than one instructor, in natural settings, where he has many opportunities to respond to natural cues and consequences.

These procedures also obviate another frequently encountered problem with moderately to severely handicapped populations. A student may learn to respond correctly for only one person, someone who has been very reinforcing with him for his appropriate behaviors. While this may be very flattering for the individual instructor, it is not in the best interests of the student since it may not result in the meaningful use of his communication and language skills. Consequently, it is important to pair yourself with at least one or two others who participate in the instruction so that he will generalize his appropriate learning behaviors to other instructors (Murdock, Garcia, & Hardman, 1977).

MATERIALS

Normally, materials will consist of all relevant stimuli, such as clothing, furniture, food, eating utensils, tools, body parts, and ongoing activities. However, there are circumstances when it is desirable and appropriate to use pictures or other representations of objects, such as when you are preparing a student to move into a more traditional educational setting. Data recording materials and tangible reinforcers (when necessary) will be required also.

HOW TO ESTABLISH COMMUNICATION AND LANGUAGE BEHAVIORS

Speech pathologists, special educators, and other professionals in the teaching and/or therapy professions are required to complete a variety of clinical methodology or educational procedures courses before they are eligible to apply for licenses or certification in their specialty areas. Normally, these courses acquaint students with a variety of techniques designed to get their future students to respond correctly to instructions or to imitate a model of the desired responses. These techniques cover a wide range and vary from what a speech pathologist may do to help his kindergarten client articulate a perfct /s/ sound to what a university professor may do to help her students understand nuclear physics.

Regardless of the age level of the student or the content of the instruction, teaching not only consists of how to reinforce or correct student responses but also of what to do in order to set the occasion for students to be able to make the initial correct response (Holland & Skinner, 1961). Consequently, there are antecedent stimuli (usually auditory and/or visual) presented to students in an attempt to arrange the environment so that they will respond correctly. This stimuli become the *discriminative stimuli* presented by instructors in order to evoke certain responses from students.

Discriminative Stimuli

Discriminative stimuli are the cues or signals which inform us that reinforcers will follow. In Chapter 2, there was considerable discussion related to how an instructor determines what is reinforcing for a particular student. Reinforcers are delivered immediately after behaviors you wish to strengthen. However, events that occur prior to student responding are also critical to learning. These events are antecedent stimuli or stimuli that you present *before* the anticipated student response, as opposed to consequent stimuli in the form of correction procedures or reinforcers delivered *after* students respond.

If these antecedent stimuli are consistently followed by reinforcing events, they become discriminative stimuli for students to respond in particular ways because they have learned that when they do so, good things follow. For example, instructors must do someting to gain students' attention at the beginning of any instructional routine. Normally, they say something like, "Watch me. Listen." This watch-me-listen signal is an excellent example of visual and auditory stimuli that have become discriminative stimuli for students to watch and listen *IF* they have been reinforced for doing so. It is obvious that this signal will not evoke desired behaviors if nothing happens or students are punished when they watch and listen.

What you say and do immediately before students respond become discriminative stimuli for them to respond in certain predictable ways, depending upon what happens afterwards. If you ask a student to match and fold her socks, and she does so, and you complement her or otherwise reinforce her for her accomplishment, she will learn to match and fold socks in response to your request because you reinforced her for doing so. On the other hand, if you make the same request and then ignore, criticize, or otherwise punish the student after she accomplished the task, she will learn not to respond to your request because she is punished for doing so (Alberto & Troutman, 1982; Axelrod, 1983; Hall, 1975; Holland & Skinner, 1961).

VARYING DISCRIMINATIVE STIMULI. Normally, multiple antecedent stimuli that represent the same concept should be presented to ensure appropriate stimulus generalization. For example, many different colors, sizes, and shapes of cups would be presented to students in order for them to learn the concept of "cup." However, moderately to severely communicatively impaired individuals frequently experience difficulty making discriminations. Therefore, for some students, it may be necessary to present very consistent antecedent stimuli when you first introduce a concept. If you are teaching "cup," you would present the same cup along with a plate, a bowl, and a spoon and say, "Hand me the cup, please." When the student can discriminate this particlar cup consistently, present a variety of cups. This may have to be done very gradually, first introducing a cup of the same size and shape but a different color, then one that differs in size and color, and finally one that differs in size, color, and shape. However, it is critical that such a wide variety of antecedent stimuli eventually be presented in order for the student to learn the concept *cupness* (Becker, Engelmann, & Thomas, 1971; Stokes & Baer, 1977). If only one exemplar is presented, such as a blue cup, the student may be discriminating on the color, not the object.

Instructing

It is obvious from the above that one of the most common teaching procedures used is to instruct students regarding what it is that you want them to do. Usually, simply instructing students is a successful procedure. Students who are under instructional control have learned that if they follow instructions, they probably will be reinforced for doing so (Hall, 1975). In other words, instructions have become discriminitive stimuli for students to respond in certain ways. Thus, it is important for *instructors* to learn that *students* will not learn to follow instructions unless they have been reinforced for doing so. Effective instructors also provide clear and concise descriptions of the behaviors they want their students to perform (Hall & Fox, 1978). Compare the following examples of two instructors who are trying to teach a student when to respond with a single word and when to use a complete sentence:

1. *Instructor:* Susan, do you remember how old you are today?
   Susan: Yes.
   Instructor: Well, how old are you?
   Susan: Twelve.
   Instructor: Susan, I don't want you to just answer the question by telling me how old you are because now we're learning how to talk in complete sentences and so I want you to use a complete sentence.
   Susan: No response.
   Instructor: That's okay, Susan. Maybe we can work on that again tomorrow.
2. *Instructor:* How old are you, Susan?
   Susan: Twelve.
   Instructor: That's right! Good answering. I can say that in a complete sentence, "I am 12 years old." Now you say it in a complete sentence, "I am 12 years old."
   Susan: I am 12 years old.
   Instructor: Right! And great answering in a complete sentence!

While the instructor in example 1 is not deliberately unkind and, in fact, probably thinks that she is being very kind to Susan, she is not presenting her instructions in a way that will lead Susan to respond correctly. First, her instructions were not clear and, second, Susan did not know when the instructor wanted a simple answer or a complete sentence. This kind of instructing not only results in students failing to have successful learning experiences but it also consumes more instructional time, which is at a premium with all student populations but particularly with moderately to severely handicapped populations.

Furthermore, and most seriously, it can teach students to respond like robots. How many moderately to severely handicapped students have you heard answer the simple question of "What is your name?" with "My name is Genevieve Elizabeth Johnson," overarticulating and prolonging every syllable, when the natural and appropriate response would have been a simple "Jenny"? The simple answer Susan gave, "Twelve," in the second example normally is the more appropriate response and she was reinforced by the second instructor for making that response. Then he modeled the complete sentence and specifically requested that Susan respond with a complete sentence. If you are teaching responding in a complete sentence, be sure to provide clear signals and only reinforce complete sentences to such simple questions as "What is your name?" or "How old are you?" in the presence of those signals and not in the presence of the questions alone (Becker, Engelmann, & Thomas, 1971). When only the questions are presented, student should be reinforced for answering with a simple "Jenny" or "Twelve."

Descriptive praise is also a very useful reinforcer in these situations because it provides additional information that tells the student exactly why she is being reinforced. Notice in example 2 above that the instructor praised Susan immediately for a right answer and he also praised her for answering in a complete sentence when those were the instructions. He might also have praised her by repeating her correct reaponse, "That's great, Susan. You said "I am 12 years old." This latter form of descriptive praise provides another model.

Modeling and Imitation

The role of modeling and imitation in language acquisition has been extremely controversial, particularly regarding its relationship to syntax (Rees, 1975). Many of the psycholinguists seem to feel that imitation has little if anything to do with learning to use language (Brown & Bellugi, 1964; Dale, 1972; Ervin, 1964; Ervin-Tripp, 1971; Slobin, 1968). On the other hand, many of the learning theorists, particularly the behaviorists, not only consider imitation to be an indispensable instructional tool, they make imitation itself an early instructional objective (Baer, Peterson, & Sherman, 1967; Guess, Sailor, Rutherford, & Baer, 1968; Lovaas, Berberich, Perloff, & Schaeffer, 1966; Sloane & MacAulay, 1968). Regardless of one's underlying philosophy regarding the role of imitation in normal language acquisition and syntax, it may be irrelevant to much of what we are talking about here in that there seems to be little or no disagreement that imitation is critical for an individual to establish and maintain functional communication (Rees, 1975). Furthermore, communication programs that use imitation as the basis for initial language acquisition have been successful, particularly with moderately to severely communicatively impaired populations (Cole & Cole, 1981; Gray & Ryan, 1973; Guess, Sailor, & Baer, 1976; Hinerman, 1983; Kent, 1974; Lovaas, 1966; Murdock & Hartmann, 1975; Striefel, 1974).

Modeling behaviors you want students to learn so that they can imitate those behaviors is a simple and effective instructional procedure (Bandura, 1969). It is simply another kind of discriminative stimuli that instructors provide for students (Hall, 1975). Notice in example 2 above that the instructor modeled the complete sentence before he asked Susan to make that response. This procedure combines clear instructions with a model of the desired response, thereby dramatically increasing the probability that Susan would respond correctly. *Always* strive to arrange instructional procedures so that students will have many successful experiences.

Most students already know how to imitate, even moderately to severely handicapped students. However, should you have a student who does not have this important skill, procedures for teaching imitation have been detailed elsewhere (see, for instance, Lovaas, 1966; Risley & Wolf, 1967; Striefel, 1974).

It is also important to provide immediate feedback to students who imitate correctly. Furthermore, other students make excellent models, particularly when instructors use descriptive praise appropriately. Consider the following example of Mr. Samuelson who is instructing Simon, Angele, Nancy, and Rod while they are eating lunch. The target behavior for all four students is to label and use a fork appropriately.

Mr. Samuelson: This is a fork. Say "fork," everybody.

Angele and Rod: Fork.

Mr. Samuelson: Great, Angele and Rod! You said, "fork." What is it, Nancy?

Nancy: Fork.

Mr. Samuelson: Wonderful! You're right. What is it, Simon?

Simon: Fork.

Mr. Samuelson Great! Watch me. I can eat with my fork. (Models the response.)

Simon immediately imitates Mr. Samuelson's model.

Mr. Samuelson: Very good, Simon! That's the way to eat with a fork.

Angele, Nancy, and Rod imitate Simon's model.

Mr. Samuelson: Hey, that's great! You can all eat with a fork.

In the above example, Mr. Samuelson was a model for all four students and both Mr. Samuelson and Simon were models for Nancy, Angele, and Rod. Mr. Samuelson accomplished this simply by modeling the eating behavior and then descriptively praising Simon's imitation. There is good evidence that individuals will be more likely to imitate a modeled behavior if they see others being reinforced for doing so (Bandura, 1969). Furthermore, the modeling and imitation were immediately functional. The students were learning the label and the function of a fork in a situation where they could immediately apply their skills.

Provide a model of any new response you are trying to teach, a response that is not presently in a student's repertoire. A model can also be presented when a student responds incorrectly. Modeling the correct response is one of the most effective prompting procedures available and can be used whenever you are not certain about what the most appropriate prompting procedure might be (Becker et al., 1971).

Prompting and Fading

A prompt is another discriminative stimuli that instructors can use to teach new behaviors. However, they are extra discriminative stimuli that are used only as needed to help students respond correctly. Only those things that a student already can do or already knows can be used as prompts (Becker et al., 1971). For example, it would be absurd to use the color of the object as a prompt to help a student locate something if the student cannot discriminate colors or to use a model as a prompt if the student cannot imitate. Generally, however, any aid an instructor provides to establish correct responding can be considered a prompt.

In the above example, Mr. Samuelson provided a fairly strong prompt because he modeled the response he was requesting. Assuming that Mr. Samuelson knows his students well, with a more advanced group of students he may have started by asking "What is this?" followed by one of the following variations of a medium prompt (Hart & Rogers-Warren, 1978): "It's a f. . ." (part of the word), or "It's not a knife, it's a . . ." (a comparison), or "It's what we use to eat green beans" (a relation). With a third group of students, he may simply have asked the question "What is this?" without providing any model.

One very important thing to keep in mind about prompting procedures is to use the weakest prompt that works because you must fade prompting procedures gradually but completely. Suggested prompting procedures to be used with this program are listed from weakest to strongest in the teaching format in Table 3-2. The same rule applies to prompts as to reinforcers: Don't do more than you have to do, but *DO* whatever is necessary (Alberto & Troutman, 1982; Axelrod, 1983; Hall, 1975; Hall & Fox, 1978; Murdock, 1978a; Murdock & Hartmann, 1975). Hall (1975) presented three major categories of prompts: verbal prompts, gestural prompts, and physical prompts.

VERBAL PROMPTS. Verbal prompts are often in the form of instructions which, if reinforced properly, can be discontinued gradually. This is particularly so when instructors set up good instructional routines. For example, there are certain behaviors that you want students to engage in routinely, such as coming into the communication and language instructional session, taking a seat, paying attention, and responding appropriately individually or with the group. When you begin working with a particular group of students, you give them all of these instructions and reinforce them for following each one as in the following example:

> *Ms. Jones:* Come here, Susan, Tim, and John.
> *Susan, Tim, and John leave what they are doing and join Ms. Jones.*
> *Ms. Jones:* Great, I like the way you come when I ask you. Sit down right here, please.
> *Susan, Tim, and John sit where Ms. Jones indicates.*
> *Ms. Jones:* Good sitting! Now, watch me, listen.
> *Susan directs her attention to Ms. Jones.*
> *Ms. Jones:* Good, you're watching me, Susan! (She pats Susan.)
> *Tim and John imitate Susan's model.*
> *Ms Jones:* Hey great, Tim and John are watching too! Now, show me what you use to eat your soup, Susan.
> *Susan picks up her spoon.*
> *Ms. Jones:* Great, Susan! What do we call this, Tim?
> *Tim:* Spoon.
> *Ms. Jones:* That's right, Tim! What do we call this, everybody?
> *Susan, Tim, and John:* Spoon.
> *Ms. Jones:* Great, you all answered!

The above is an example of instructions given on the first day. It's obvious that a instructor will not continue to repeat and reinforce appropriate responding to these preliminary instructions because it is not necessary. These instructions can be faded out gradually because students learn that certain behaviors are expected by instructors in certain situations and, once they learn to discriminate and understand the routine, they will continue to respond appropriately for as long as they are reinforced for doing so.

GESTURAL PROMPTS. In the above example, gestures were a natural part of the communication process. However, they also served as additional cues or as prompts. Ms. Jones motioned with her hand as she said "Come here." She pointed to chairs around the lunch table as she said "Sit down, please." She used gestures as she said "Watch me. Listen." She patted Susan when she praised her for watching, thus using Susan as a model for good attending behaviors and letting Tim and John see that imitating attending would probably be reinforced.

Ms. Jones also employed other good instructional procedures. For example, she paused strategically in order to hold the students' attention (Becker et al., 1971). It is particularly important to pause before saying a student's name and to say the name *after* you have asked the question or given the instruction; otherwise, other students in the group may not attend to the question or instruction because they know they will not be asked to respond (Becker et al., 1971).

PHYSICAL PROMPTS. If verbal and gestural prompts fail to establish the desired response, use physical prompts. Physical prompting varies from slightly touching a student to physically taking him through the desired response. While it is not usually feasible to physically prompt speaking, there are many communicative behaviors that can be prompted physically, such as gestures and signs. The following steps are adapted from Striefel (1974) and are used for systematically prompting and fading a gesture which communicates that the student is thirsty.

1. Define the target behavior: On the request, "What do you want?" the student is to raise his preferred hand to his lips as though holding a glass.
2. Provide a model which would normally occasion the behavior: When you know that the student has been without water or other fluids for some time, place a glass of water in front of him and make the request "What do you want?" Seat the student facing you with hands on knees and say, "Raise your hand to your lips."
3. If the student does not respond correctly, repeat the discriminative stimuli "What do you want?" and physically guide the student through the response as you say, "Raise your hand to your lips," while grasping the student's preferred hand, forming it as though the student were holding a glass, and raising it to the student's lips.
4. Verbally reinforce the student immediately after the prompted response by saying "Great!" or whatever you choose, paired with a social reinforcer such as a hug, a pat, or a handshake, and give him some of the water.
5. Repeat this procedure at least three or four times or until you do not feel the student resisting your physical prompting.
6. Now begin fading the physical prompts by guiding the student through all but the very last step of the behavior, being sure to reinforce him for completing the response. Say, "What do you want? Raise your hand to your lips," grasping his hand and guiding it to a 3/4 raised position, letting him complete the last part of the hand raise alone. Reinforce immediately with social consequences and some water.
7. Continue fading by guiding the student through less and less of the response. Say "What do you want? Raise your hand to your lips," while grasping his hand and guiding him through 2/3, then 1/2, 1/3, 1/4, 1/8 of the hand-raising response.
8. Continue fading the physical prompts until you are merely touching his

hand, then merely making a gesture toward him as he begins to make the response. Say "What do you want?" while gesturing toward his hand and letting him complete the response. Reinforce immediately with social consequences and water.

9. Fade out the gesture so that the student is making the response without prompts. Say "What do you want?" Let him make the response without prompts. Reinforce immediately with social consequences and water.
10. Continue reinforcing each correct response until the communicative gesture is well established.

Chaining

So far, we have discussed behaviors as though each behavior were an independent act. Actually, each behavior is a complex set of simpler responses that, combined, comprise what is called a *chain* or a *behavioral chain* (Alberto & Troutman, 1982; Axelrod, 1983; Hall, 1975; Hall & Fox, 1978; Panyon, 1975). In the example of Ms. Jones in the section on "Prompting and Fading," Ms. Jones was presenting discriminative stimuli in the form of requests and reinforcing every appropriate response the students made, or, to put it another way, she was reinforcing every link in the chain. Eventually, however, each link in the chain serves as the discriminative stimuli for the next response, and the reinforcer is delivered at the end of the chain. When this has been accomplished, the above example of Ms. Jones instructing her students would be as follows:

Ms. Jones: Come here, Susan, Tim, and John.
Susan, Tim, and John leave what they are doing and join Ms. Jones.
They sit appropriately without being requested to do so.
Ms. Jones: Watch me. Listen. Show me what you use to eat your soup, Susan.
Susan picks up her spoon.
Ms. Jones: Great, Susan! What do we call this, Tim?
Tim: Spoon
Ms. Jones: Good, Tim. What do we call this, everybody?
Susan, Tim and John: Spoon.
Ms. Jones: Wonderful, you all answered!

As you can see, Ms. Jones no longer needs to reinforce the students for coming to her upon request. Nor does she need to instruct the students to sit down and then reinforce them for doing so. Nor does she need to reinforce Susan for attending, thus using her as a model for Tim and John. Nor does she need to reinforce Tim and John for finally attending. She only had to do this initially until she had established this behavioral chain in which Susan, Tim, and John had learned that each step in the chain was the discriminative stimuli for the next response, with reinforcers only being provided at the end of the coming-to-session-and-paying-attention routine when Susan correctly identified the spoon.

The above is an example of forward chaining. When teaching communication and language skills, it is sometimes more efficient to use a backward chaining approach. In a backward chain, you teach the last link in the chain first, then the next to the last link, and so on until, finally, the initial link is mastered. Mr. Kelly has a student named Felicia who has many single words in her vocabulary but who does not combine words. Mr. Kelly decides to use a backward chaining procedure because it is much easier for him to present the visual discriminative stimuli for a word like "milk" than it is for words like "I" and "want" to form the sentence "I want milk." Furthermore, Felicia can already respond correctly with the word "milk" when it is designated and she is requested to do so. The backward chaining procedure to accomplish the above would be as follows:

> *Mr. Kelly:* I want milk. How about you, Felicia? What do you want? (pointing to a glass about one quarter full of the milk).
> *Felicia:* Milk.
> *Mr. Kelly:* Good! You said, "milk." (Gives her some milk.) I can say the whole sentence, "I want milk." Now you say the whole sentence. What do you want? (Offers milk.) Say "I want ____."
> *Felicia:* Milk
> *Mr. Kelly:* Great, you finished the sentence, Felicia! (Gives her some more milk.) What do you want, Felicia? (Offers milk.) Say the whole sentence. "I *want* ____." ("I" is said softly and "want" is said loudly.)
> *Felicia:* Milk.
> *Mr. Kelly:* Say the whole sentence, Felicia. What do you want? Say "I *want* ____." (Stressed "want" again.)
> *Felicia:* Wan' milk.
> *Mr. Kelly:* Wonderful, Felicia! (Gives her some more milk.) You're learning to say, "I want milk." Say the whole sentence again. What do you want? (Offers milk.) Say "*I want* ____." (Both "I" and "want" are stressed.)
> *Felicia:* Milk.
> *Mr. Kelly:* Say the whole sentence, Felicia. What do you want? (Still offering milk.) Say "*I want* ____." (Both "I" and "want" receive stress.)
> *Felicia:* Want milk.
> *Mr. Kelly:* Good, Felicia! (Gives her some more milk.) Let's say the whole sentence again. What do you want? (Offering milk.) Say "*I* want ____." (Only "I" is stressed.)
> *Felicia:* I want milk.
> *Mr. Kelly:* Beautiful, Felicia! (Gives her some more milk.) Say the whole sentence again. What do you want? (Offers milk.) Say "I want ____."

("Want" is almost whispered.)

Felicia: I want milk.

Mr. Kelly: Fantastic, Felicia! (Gives her some more milk.) You can say the whole sentence. Let's do it again. What do you want? (offers milk.) Say "I ____ ____."

Felicia: I want milk.

Mr. Kelly: You're wonderful! (Gives her some more milk.) Let's say the whole sentence again. What do you want? (Offers milk.)

Felicia: I want milk.

Mr. Kelly: That's fantastic! (Gives her the remainder of the milk.) Let's go ask Ms. Anderson for some more milk.

Notice how Mr. Kelly shifted the criteria for responses that he would reinforce. Once Felicia said "Wan' milk," he no longer reinforced her when she responded with just "Milk." In this sense chaining is very similar to shaping. Mr. Kelly consistently repeated the request to speak in a complete sentence and the question "What do you want?" while offering Felicia milk. These procedures are not without controversy because they detract from natural narrative. However, this is an example of establishing a chain of behaviors that is not presently in the student's verbal repertoire. Therefore, very consistent antecedent stimuli were presented to signal the student how and when to respond. As was pointed out in the preceding section on "Discriminative Stimuli," when correct responding is established, antecedent stimuli must be varied until they become those used in natural discourse. Varying antecedent stimuli is also important for generalization, which will be discussed in Chapter 5.

Notice at the conclusion of this training segment, Mr. Kelly said, "Let's go ask Ms. Anderson for some more milk." This entire training segment provides a basis for the concept of *more* and will be used by Mr. Kelly (or others) later on adding the word *more* to the sentence, teaching Felicia to say, "I want more (milk)."

Shaping

Both chaining and shaping are procedures used to establish new behaviors. Perhaps the most important distinction between the two is that chaining normally is used to link already existing behaviors (as in the above example where Felica was already able to produce each of the words in the chain separately) and shaping is used to develop a new form of behavior, beginning with the closest approximation to that form that is already in the student's behavioral repertoire (Axelrod, 1983; Panyon, 1975; Sloane, Johnston, & Harris, 1968). When a behavior does not occur or it occurs at a very low frequency, and instructing or modeling fail, shaping procedures are necessary in order to establish the behavior (Hall & Fox, 1978). Shaping is a procedure which involves differentially reinforcing successive approximations to the desired behavior (Holland & Skinner, 1961). This process involves reinforcing behaviors that progressively resemble the desired target behavior.

Begin by identifying any behavior the student exhibits that is even remotely related to the target behavior. Select a behavior that the student performs readily in order to ensure a maximum of successful experiences, at least initially. When this initial behavior occurs consistently in response to the discriminative stimuli you are presenting, gradually shift your expectations for responses that will be reinforced, just as Mr. Kelly did in the session on "Chaining." Shift again, when the second behavior occurs consistently, and so forth, until the student is reinforced only for exhibiting the target behavior (Alberto & Troutman, 1982; Axelrod, 1983; Hall, 1975; Hall & Fox, 1978; Holland & Skinner, 1961; Murdock, 1978a; Panyon, 1975; Sloane & MacAulay, 1968).

In the following example, Ms. Garcia is using a shaping procedure to teach her student Al to say "hi."

Ms. Garcia: Hi, Al. Say "hi."

Al appears to attend but does not open his mouth or say anything.

Ms. Garcia: Hi, Al. Say "hi."

Al opens his mouth.

Ms. Garcia: Good, you're trying to say "hi," Al! (Gives him some apple juice.) Try it again. Say "hi."

Al opens his mouth and there is a slight aspiration.

Ms. Garcia: Wonderful! (She gives him some apple juice.) You're learning to say "hi." Let's try it again. Say "hi."

Al: Huuuh.

Ms. Garcia: Fantastic! (She gives him some apple juice and strokes his cheek.) Let's do it again. Say "hi."

Al: Huuh.

Ms. Garcia: Good. You're doing fine, Al. (She pats him.) Let's try it again. Say "hi."

Al: Hai.

Ms. Garcia: Fantastic, Al! (She pats him and gives him some juice.) You can do it again. Say "hi."

Al: Hi.

Ms. Garcia: You've got it, Al! That's wonderful! (She gives him some apple juice and strokes his cheek.) Let's hear it again. Say "hi."

Al: Huh.

Ms. Garcia: No, Al. I want to hear "hi." You can do it. Watch me (moves hand with apple juice slightly below her mouth). Listen. Say "hi."

Al: Hi.

Ms. Garcia: Fantastic! I told you you could do it. (Pats him.) Again. Say "hi."

Al: Hi.

Ms. Garcia: You're wonderful! (Gives him some apple juice and pats him.) One more time, Al. Say "hi."

Al: Hi.

Ms. Garcia: You've got it! Come on, let's go say "hi" to Mr. Kelly.

Notice how Ms. Garcia only reinforced those responses that were better approximations to the target behavior "hi." She made the determaination that "hai" was closer than "huuh." Therefore, once Al responded with "hai," "huuh" was not reinforced. By providing such differential reinforcement, only reinforcing those responses that Al made that most closely approximated the target behavior of saying "hi," Al learned to produce the new response.

How to Establish Specific Language Structures

The provisions set forth in CLIP for assessing communication and language skills by taking spontaneous communication and language samples and for delivering instruction in natural environments are intended to ensure that students will be taught the semantic and pragmatic rules that are appropriate to their particular language community. However, speech-language pathologists, teachers, and parents we have worked with frequently have requested some guidelines regarding what phonological, syntactic, and morphological structures to teach and how to establish those structures. This section is included in response to those requests.

Phonological Structures

With moderately to severely communicatively impaired populations, simple articulation problems generally are low priority. However, a phonological disorder may exist with this population that is not a simple articulation disorder but, on closer examination, reveals frequent syllable omission and inconsistent use of functors (i.e., form words such as articles, prepositions, conjunctions, and auxiliary verbs which mark grammatical structure and modify meaning). Thus, the disorder becomes both semantic and morphological in nature. When a student is very difficult to understand, the instructor may select specific words in his environment to teach him to say more clearly. It is helpful to consider the sequence in which normal children learn to say particular phonemes or sounds. This sequence can be thought of as beginning with generally easier sounds and ending with those that are more difficult to produce. Easier sounds appear to be those shaped by large movements of the lips, tongue, and jaw (e.g., vowel sounds). Usually, visible sounds are easier to produce (e.g., b, p, m, d, and t). However, some phonemes that are visible are more difficult to produce because they require finer motor coordination (e.g., l, f, v, and th/). Sounds that are a combination of two sounds are also more difficult to produce (e.g., d and zh = j; t and sh = ch). Consonant sounds that appear in a string (st, gl, str, etc.) are also more difficult to produce. Based on Sanders's (1972) norms, the following sequence is the order in which sounds are learned by normal children: n, m, p, h, t, k, f, w, ng, b, g, s, y, d, l, r, sh, ch, j, v, s, zh, and th.

These students need to learn the rules for combining sound symbols with morphemes. According to Lucas (1980), modeling patterns of morphophonemic rules for the students to imitate is usually a more effective teaching procedure than working on specific sounds. In addition to modeling, it may also be useful to use some of the instructional, prompting, shaping, and chaining procedures described above.

Syntactic and Morphological Structures

Table 3-1 provides examples of syntactic and morphological structures normally acquired by children who are 3½ or 4 years old along with suggestions for establishing these structures. Table 3-2 is a sample teaching format that corresponds to Table 3-1. These tables can be used as models for any communication and language skill that you are teaching.

TABLE 3-1

SYNTACTIC (WORD ORDER) AND MORPHOLOGICAL (WORD FORM) STRUCTURES

The following list is not a complete developmental sequence but is a teaching sequence which should result in pragmatic communication involving up to five- to seven-word utterances.

The structures within each stage are not listed in any particular order unless specifically noted.

Note the normal telegraphic use of content (critical) words in Stages A, B and C.

(There are no *specific* norms for these expressive language skills.)

Stage A: Two-Word Utterances — Pivots*

Intent†	*Examples*‡ (Student)	*Possible Questions* (If Silence and the Situation Don't Work) (Instructor)
Something exists! (Person or object appears.)	• *There* ball. *There* cookie. *That* ball. *That* cookie. *Hi* puppy. *Hi* Mommy.	What's going on? *or* What happened?
Something reoccurs. (Show or offer more of same thing.)	• *More* ball, *More* cookie. *'Nother* cookie. *'Nother* car.	What's going to happen?
Three uses of negatives:		
• Something isn't there or disappears	• *No* ball. *No* cookie. Ball *all gone.*	What do you say? etc.
• Rejection (Offer something student doesn't like.)	• *No* carrot! *No* go. *Bye-bye* carrot. *Bye-bye* Pat.	
• Denial (Describe something incorrectly.)	• *No* horsie! *No* milk! *No* good! (Last negative to appear.)	

*Pivot structures contain one frequently used word combined with many other words which are usually nouns. Each pivot word can take eaither the first or second position.

†A student's intent can often be discovered by watching the gestures occurring when she makes an utterance.

‡Change of intonation can make the same structure function as a comment, a request or a question.

Table 3-1 (Continued)

Stage B: Two-Word Utterances — Pivot Plus

Intent	*Sturcture**	*Examples* (Student)	*Possible Questions* (Instructor)
Action + object	V + N	Throw ball. Read book.	• What should (person) do? What is(person) doing?
Agent + action	N + V	Mommy throw. Mommy read.	• What's happening? What's going to happen?
Agent + object	N + N	Mommy bread. Dog bowl.	• What did Mommy do? What do you see?
Possession	N + N	Mommy coat. My cookie.	• Whose cookie is this? What's this? (Must ask both.)
Location	V (or) N + N	Go store. Mommy store.	• Where did Mommy go? What happened to Mommy? (Must ask both.)
Description	Adj + N	Big ball. Two cookie.	• What about this cookie? What's this?
Question	Wh-?	What that? Where go?	

Key:
*V = verb = action word, N = noun = name of something, Adj = adjective = descriptive word, Prep = preposition = location.

Stage C: Three-Word Utterances

	Structure	*Examples* (Student)	*Possible Questions* (Instructor)
Word Order:	N + V + N	Mommy read book. Daddy wash dishes.	What's (person) doing?
	V + N + Location	Put baby bed. Put cookie there.	What's happening?
	N + Adj + N (Possession)	Mom pretty dress. Doggy big bowl.	What's this?
	V + Prep + N	Go in car. Hide under chair.	How did Daddy go? What's the doggy doing?
	V + Adj + N	See big ball. Spill purple juice.	What do you see? What happened?
	(Person) + no + V	Daddy no go. I no sleep.	How about (person)?
	can't don't	I can't go. Don't go store.	What do you want to do?
	where what	Where Mom go? What Bobby eat?	What do you want to know?
Word Form:	+ ing	Baby sleeping. Going bye-bye.	What's happening?
	+ s (plural)	I want cookies. The big dogs.	What do you want? What do you see?

Table 3-1 (Continued)

me my I	Cookie in me. My new coat. I want more.	Where did it go? What about this?
the a an	In the box. Want a cookie. Want an apple.	Where is it? I want a cookie, how about you?

Stage D: Three- to Four-Word Utterances

	Structure	*Examples* (Student)	*Possible Questions* (Instructor)
Word Order:	N + is* + Adj	Daddy's mad. The water is dirty.	How about (person or thing)?
	N + is + Verb + ing	Mommy's working. The dog is eating.	What's happening? What is (person or thing) doing?
	gonna hafta can will	You gonna go. I hafta go. I can run. I'll do it.	What's going to happen? What's happening?
	won't didn't isn't	Didn't go home. I won't go. This isn't mine.	What's going on? What about this?
	are is	Is he going, too? Are they ready now?	What do you want to know?
	what where who	What is it? Who is it? Where you going?	What do you want to know?
Word Form:	+ s† (possession)	It's Mom's coat. Is it Mary's?	Whose coat is that?
	he she they them	He is wet. She's nice. They're happy. Give it to them.	How about (person or thing)?

*The contracted form, /'s/, often appears first in the majority of occurrences. If a student's sound production does not include a final /s/, it will be difficult to know if the student is indeed marking *is* with /'s/ in fast speech. When this occurs, the instructor's models should have *is* in its noncontracted form.
†This may not be possible for a student who does not have the final /s/.

Stage E: Four- to Five-Word Utterances

	Structure	*Examples* (Student)	*Possible Questions* (Instructor)
Word Order:	N + are + adj	They are too tired. My shoes are all wet.	What about (person or thing?)
	N + are + verb + ing	The dogs are barking. We're going right now.	What's happening?
	can will do (questions)	Can I have some? Will you give me some? Do you live here?	What do you want to know? How do you ask?
Word Form:	V + S (States of body, emotion, or habitual activity)	She likes hugs and kisses. She always breaks my toys.	What does (person or thing) always do?
	V + ed	Mommy kissed it better. I picked up my clothes.	What happend with Mommy? Who picked up your clothes?
	we	We're going home. We have to go now.	What about you and (person or thing)?

Table 3-1 (Continued)

Stage F; Five- to Seven-Word Utterances

Structure	*Examples* (Student)	*Possible Questions* (Instructor)
N + was + adj or V	My Mom was tired last night . . . Janie was sleeping in the car.	What happened? What was (person or thing) doing?
N + were + Adj or V	The kids were mean to me. The kids were shouting too much.	What happened with those (people or things)?
because if so and	I'm crying because I'm sad. I'll go if you do. I ate mine, so you eat yours. I ate mine and you eat yours.	Why are you crying? What do you mean? Why do you want (person or thing) to do that?
when won't wasn't	When are we going to go? Won't he do his work Wasn't she sick yesterday?	What do you want to know?

TABLE 3-2

SAMPLE TEACHING FORMAT FOR SYNTACTIC AND MORPHOLOGICAL STRUCTURES

Establish baselines as described in Chapter 4 before beginning intervention. When using this format, begin by presenting number 3 in the first column (Verbal) ten times. Then move sequentially from number 1 through number 4.

Discriminative Stimuli (Instructor)				
(1) Verbal	(2) Visual	(3) Prompts to Be Used Only If Needed	(4) Response (Student)	(5) Consequent Stimuli (Instructor)
1. Ask appropriate question* and then use structure two times providing answer, e.g., "What do you think about this apple? The apple is red. The apple is good."	Activities with objects or pictures.	Listed from weakest to strongest prompt. Pause before difficult part of structure as it occurs in your model. Auditorily exaggerate difficult parts of the structure. Visually and auditorily exaggerate the difficult parts of the structure. Say difficult parts of the structure with the student.	Correct response (Two responses in step 3) (Articulation errors made on phenomes not previously trained are acceptable.)	Listed from strongest to weakest reinforcers. CRF Social CRF Tangible CRF Social FR 2 Tangible CRF Social VR 3 Tangible
2. Provide three to five models of structure and then ask appropriate questions e.g., "This apple is red. This apple is good. What do you think?"		Say entire structure with the student. Say entire structure with the student while holding her arm or hand and moving it in rhythm with the words. Shape the structure.		CRF Social VR 5 Tangible

*Appropriate questions are listed as part of Figure 3-1, Syntactic and Morphological Structures.

Table 3-2 (Continued)

(1) Verbal	(2) Visual	(3) Prompts to Be Used Only If Needed	(4) Response (Student)	(5) Consequent Stimuli (Instructor)
3. Provide multiple models appropriate to structure and the student's activity. Rarely infer need for response by asking questions. Say, "The apple is red. The apple is good." (Wait for response from student.) 4. Ask appropriate questions only if silence and the situation aren't adequate to stimulate the response. When working on morphological forms, proceed through steps 1 to 4 above with morpheme(s) in sentence.			Incorrect response	No reinforcer. Repeat, adding prompt.

GENERAL DIRECTIONS FOR USING THE SAMPLE TEACHING FORMAT. The sample teaching format provides an easy-to-follow guide regarding how to gradually fade out the prompts completely and reduce the tangible reinforcers you give a student until they are also completely eliminated. The data recording procedures described in Chapter 4 and the graphs you keep of these data will clearly indicate when a student has mastered any particular task so that you can use it as a review item to be interspersed with new, more difficult tasks.

Criteria for progression in each column of Table 3-1 are five consecutive correct responses or 80 percent or better correct responding for two consecutive sessions, or whatever criteria the communication and language instructor deems appropriate. These may vary considerably from student to student. Each time a student reaches the predetermined criteria on any particular task, the order of movement in Table 3-2, the teaching format, is as follows:

1. Columns 1 and 2 provide verbal and visual discriminative stimuli presented by the instructor. They are listed in a teaching sequence from most structured to least-structured (easiest to most difficult). Use the least-structured antecedent discriminative stimuli that result in correct responding. As a student reaches criteria, move to progressively less-structured discriminative stimuli. (Indicate the discriminative stimuli you are using on the data recording sheet.)
2. Column 3 lists prompts, which are also antecedent discriminative stimuli that can be presented by the instructor. They are listed from weakest to strongest. Use a prompt only if a student does not respond correctly without prompting. If a prompt is required, use the weakest prompt that will result in correct responding. As a student reaches criteria, move to progressively weaker prompts. Fade prompts in column 3 until the student can respond correctly without being prompted. (Indicate the prompt to be used on the data recording sheet.)
3. Column 4 is included to help the instructor stay aware of the necessity of defining an acceptable response from the student, that is, one that will be reinforced.
4. Column 5 lists the reinforcement schedules from strongest to weakest (most to least dense). Start with the strongest, that is, reinforce every correct response. When the student has mastered the task without prompting, move progressively down this column, thinning the reinforcement schedule until you are only reinforcing about every fifth correct response (VR 5 reinforcement schedule). (Indicate the reinforcement schedule you are using on your data recording sheet.)
5. When the student has mastered a task without any prompting and is on a VR 5 reinforcement schedule, the task becomes a review task. Review tasks are particularly useful to intersperse when students are experiencing considerable failure. Such interspersion guarantees a high success rate.

ADDITIONAL NOTES ABOUT TEACHING SYNTACTIC AND MORPHOLOGICAL STRUCTURES. When you are teaching syntactic or morphological structures, you aren't teaching sentences or words, you're teaching *rules*. For example, when you teach a student about using "action-object" structures, you teach him the rule that: *First you say the action word (or verb) and* then *the object is acted upon.* More important, you teach by examples. To teach a rule, it is important to provide a student with *several examples* of that rule (e.g., "This is Mom's purse," "These are Anthony's boots," and "That's Celia's dessert"). Examples such as these are given to teach the morphological rule which is concerned with the possessive / + s/ in Table 3-1.

Consider also presenting examples to teach a student to use a verb phrase: "Throw the ball," "Roll the ball, "Kick the ball," etc. Note that in the examples, or models, of these structures, the complete, not telegraphic, phrase using *the* is given. The *student* may respond in *his* own telegraphic way with, "Throw ball," with*out* the article *the*. It is our experience that the student will use the parts of the instructor's model that are possible for him to use at his stage of language development. The instructor's models must be short enough for the student to process but are rarely telegraphic. Normally, they should expose the student to correct short but complete examples of the structure. The student's usual longest length of utterance can be used as a guide for choosing the length of the instructor's models. For example, if a student does not say more than four to five words in an utterance, it would be best to make the models of, for example, *is* questions short: "Is it hot?" or "Is the soup ready?" as opposed to "Is the soup that's on the kitchen stove ready or is it still too cold?" which is too long.

When you are selecting models of the structure you are teaching, fit them into a comment, question, or direction which relates to what the student is interested in and/or doing at the moment. For example, if you are teaching the morphological form *he* and the student is playing with the Sesame Street dolls Bert and Ernie in a tub of water, you could say, "*He* wants to swim" and "*He* wants to splash." If the student takes the dolls out of the water and puts them under a towel, you would then say, "*He's* getting dry" and "*He's* hiding." Follow the student's immediate interest. It's important to use the same structure in many different situations and, therefore, different sentences by just shifting the vocabulary. Your models should fit naturally into the activity of the moment.

A variety in your vocal inflections and vocabulary is also important so that the student (and you) don't get bored and so that he is indeed learning a rule, not just a specific sentence. To make the use of two or three models seem more natural, sometimes you may add surprise, question, or other inflection to your model. You might give the student a choice, with one of your examples being more accurate than the other. For example, "The apple is red? The apple is green." (The apple is indeed red.) It is also enjoyable for some students if one of your models is wrong or silly, "The apple is red? The apple is blue." It is helpful to make the last model declarative with a downward inflection. This prevents the student from learning to say a structure with a predominantly upward, question inflection.

As mentioned earlier, appropriate intonation, loudness, and inflection patterns are important in your models, just as they are in the student's responses. You may need to emphasize a part of a model in order to prompt the student's correct response, but be sure to return to a natural model as soon as the student has mastered the form and, ultimately, reinforce only natural prosody.

Except when using chaining or shaping procedures as described above, avoid adding pitch or loudness change to emphasize a structure. Attempt to make the target structure more prominent by the use of pauses, such as "The apple (pause) is (pause) red."

The variety of vocabulary in your models should be *controlled* when a target structure is first introduced. If all the parts of a sentence are changed in each model, it may distract a student from the structure she is to hear. For example, during the early teaching of a structure, it would be more appropriate to model, "It's Dad'*s* (pause) coat. It's Mom'*s* coat? No, it's Dad'*s* coat."

More variety in the models would be appropriate in the latter stages of learning a structure. An illustration of more variety in the instructor's models would be: "Where's Dad'*s* coat? Let's find Mom'*s* boots and Roberto'*s* mittens too. I can't reach Jennifer'*s* scarf."

Appropriate questions are suggested for each syntactic and morphological structure in Table 3-1. They are geared to make the full and correct response likely to occur. They avoid "short-answer" questions which are so often used with students and which result in responses other than the target structure. For example, if you are teaching the use of /+ed/ to indicate past tense in sentences, when you ask the student the short-answer question, "What did Grover do?" he'll very logically respond, "Jump" or, possibly, "Jumped." But if you use an appropriate question, such as, "What's happened here?" or "What's with Grover?" the student will very likely respond, "Grover jumped" or "He jumped." It is better if it isn't necessary to ask the student a question. A little silence or the situation itself may be enough to stimulate the student's response. On step 3, it is most effective to provide just models that would trigger the student's response. For example, the instructor might make a ridiculous statement, thus providing a cue for the student to make the correction. While on step 3, the student may not respond until she has heard many models from the instructor. She is learning by listening to models describing what she is immediately watching or doing. The need for her to respond is only *inferred.* She is not required to respond on this step.

On step 4, the student is required to take conversational turns. If she does not respond, the instructor should wait for up to 5 or 10 seconds and then infer nonverbally that the student should respond by looking at her, gesturing, or saying "Your turn." If the student doesn't respond, the instructor should provide another model and again infer that she should respond.

Only if such natural language intervention procedures fail is it necessary to use precise shaping procedures in an attempt to teach a student morphology and syntax. These shaping procedures would entail either forward or backward chaining. It has been our experience that backward chaining is more effective. However, again, be responsive to how the particular student you are working with responds.

Using one of the examples from above in a chaining procedure, you would say, "What happened with Grover? (pause) He jumped." You may need to talk in unison with the student, moving his hand in rhythm with the words. If the student does not respond appropriately, you would say, "What did Grover do? Jumped." When this response becomes stable in this isolated form, that is, he responds "Jumped" at 80 percent or better for two consecutive teaching sessions, then you would ask, "What happened with Grover? He jumped." Then only reinforce "He jumped" or "Grover jumped." By altering the question, you can avoid saying, "Say 'He jumped'" and still get short and then longer responses.

Where the full form of a structure is presented, some students may respond with the contracted form. For example, when a student hears, "He is sleeping," he may respond with, "He's sleeping." It is appropriate to reinforce the student for either of these grammatical forms which are both correct. When a student's preference for one of these forms (either the full or the contracted form) is shown, we have found it effective to then model using that form.

To summarize, the important procedures to remember when teaching syntactic and morphological structures are:

1. Present *two or more examples or models* of the structure or form you're teaching on steps 1 and 2 before the student responds. On step 3, provide multiple models not requiring a response. On step 4, provide one model while taking conversational turns.
2. Say the functors or little words that are part of a *complete,* if short, example of the structure.
3. The length of your models should fit the student's ability to respond.
4. Let your models describe or ask about what the student is *actively* and *currently* interested or involved in.
5. *Vary* the inflection of your voice and the vocabulary changes only slightly so the student can attend to the target structure.
6. At first vary the vocabulary changes only slightly so the student can attend to the target structure.
7. Use *natural stress* in your examples or models except when it is necessary to use chaining or shaping procedures. Use pauses as prompts only if they are needed.

8. Be sure the questions you ask are answerable *logically* by the structure you are teaching.
9. Whenever possible, let a little *silence* or the *situation* trigger the student's response.
10. Precise chaining or shaping procedures are used only in cases where a student fails to respond appropriately in a variety of situations that were arranged to evoke correct syntax and morphology. In these instances, use appropriate questions and shorter units of models and responses to teach the correct structure.

HOW TO MAINTAIN AND STRENGTHEN COMMUNICATION AND LANGUAGE BEHAVIORS

Reinforcement

As discussed in Chapter 2, by definition, a reinforcer maintains or strengthens the behavior it follows. In order to keep or strengthen the communication and language behaviors established through instructing, modeling, prompting, or shaping procedures, you must reinforce them. This section covers different types of reinforcers, what to reinforce, when to reinforce, how to reinforce, and reinforcement schedules.

Types of Reinforcers

NATURAL REINFORCERS. A natural reinforcer is anything that normally occurs in a particular environment that strengthens behaviors it follows. There are many naturally occurring reinforcers in home, school, and community environments. Unfortunately, many of them are wasted. Or worse, they are delivered immediately after inappropriate behaviors, thus strengthening those inappropriate behaviors.

For example, there are television sets in most homes and in many classrooms. An individual who disrupts ongoing family or classroom routines by giggling and flapping her hands is often removed from the situation and placed in front of a television, which keeps her occupied and out of trouble and allows parents or instructors to continue whatever they are doing. However, in all probability, watching television is a reinforcing activity that will strengthen or increase the rate of the removed individual's disruptive behaviors. Arrange environments so that naturally occurring reinforcers only strengthen *appropriate* behaviors. In the above example, a brief time-out from any reinforcers would have been a better choice. Later on, contingent upon not giggling and keeping her hands folded in lap except when pointing or making other communicative gestures, the timed-out individual could watch some television.

Use natural reinforcers whenever it is possible because they are (1) readily available, (2) usually less expensive, (3) usually less trouble to arrange, and (4) much more likely to be available and presented by other individuals who have contact with the students (Hall, 1975; Hall & Fox, 1978).

SOCIAL REINFORCERS. Social reinforcers, including verbal praise, are very desirable reinforcers to use, not only because they are natural in school, at home and in community environments, but also because the student is not as likely to satiate on social consequences as on edible reinforcers, for instance. Furthermore, social consequences do not result in cavities, obesity or hyperactivity as do many of the edible reinforcers.

Examples of verbal praise might be, "I like the way you said 'Mama.' That was fantastic!" or "You really know how to say the whole sentence, Janie! Good talking!" Such descriptive praise lets the student know exactly what she is being reinforced for and, consequently, is a very desirable reinforcer (Becker et al., 1971). Physical contact is another social reinforcer. This might be shaking hands, patting on the head, stroking her cheek or chin, hugging or tickling. Smiling and eye contact also serve as social reinforcers.

ACTIVITY REINFORCERS. Activities that the student prizes can also be used as reinforcers (Premack, 1959). Frequently, instructors observe activities that are reinforcing for a particular student during the preprogram observations. Activities like social reinforcers are highly desirable because the student is not so likely to satiate and they are natural to classroom, home, and community environments. However, it may be more difficult to deliver an activity reinforcer immediately, in which case you should reinforce the student with verbal praise, letting her know that the activity is coming up later. If this does not prove successful, immediately deliver tokens or some other tangible reinforcer that later can be traded for the upcoming activity (Hall, 1975; Hall & Fox, 1978).

TANGIBLE PRIMARY REINFORCERS. Tangible reinforcers might be token or primary reinforcers. Primary reinforcers are anything the student can eat or drink. It is often necessary with very young and/or very handicapped students to use tangible reinforcers. And, at least initially, it is often necessary to use primary reinforcers.

In order to minimize satiation, give the student very small bits of food. We have found that a tiny bit of banana or a small taste of apple sauce, for example, is just as effective and generally more desirable than large pieces of chocolate candy or a lot of sugar-coated cereal. A taste of fruit juice delivered either with a spoon or squirted directly into the child's mouth is also very effective. The fruit juice can be put in a regular plastic bottle with a nozzle tip such as one used to tint hair. These can be washed along with the regular dishes or put into the dishwasher. Not only is this an efficient way to deliver a primary rienforcer, but it is also very novel for most students. Novelty in and of itself can be reinforcing (Hall, 1975). Remember to thin the reinforcement schedule so that you are reinforcing intermittently as soon as possible. Not only does this reduce the satiation problem, but it makes the behaviors much more persistent and more likely to remain in the student's repertoire when they are no longer being reinforced deliberately.

Whatever edible reinforcer you select, it should not be something that takes a long time to chew or swallow because this interferes with many of the communication and language behaviors that you are trying to teach, particularly talking. This is another reason for giving very small bites. Use the natural environment by teaching names of foods and eating utensils, as well as other language behaviors, during snacktime and lunchtime when the student can receive bites of her food for responding correctly.

Always pair social consequences such as praise, smiles, hugs, pats, etc., with tangible edible reinforcers so that the social consequences will eventually become just as reinforcing as food or beverages. Therefore, the food or beverages can eventually be faded out completely except when they would occur naturally.

TANGIBLE TOKEN REINFORCERS. Tokens are like money in our society, and in order to be effective, they must provide a means for the student to buy something that he wants. Tokens can be anything tangible that you give the student that later can be traded in for a backup reinforcer in order to strengthen desirable behaviors.

Select tokens that will not interfere with ongoing teaching. A token that the student attends to rather than attending to you is not an effective reinforcer. We have found that placing the "+'s" on the data recording sheet can be effective tokens if they're backed up with something the student wants, such as food, a prize, an activity, etc. (Murdock & Sabrio, 1983).

Tokens are useful because they are something tangible that you can deliver immediately and easily, yet you do not have to be as concerned about nutrition and satiation as you are when you're using primary reinforcers. However, it may be necessary to establish tokens as reinforcers when you're working with severely handicapped students or with young children who have not learned that money or other forms of tokens have value. When this occurs, it is necessary to consistently associate or pair the tokens with primary reinforcers or other previously conditioned reinforcers. The same principle is involved as with pairing primary reinforcers with social consequences. You want the tokens to become conditioned or secondary reinforcers that take on the same reinforcing properties as the primary reinforcers. Otherwise, they're simply neutral events for the student and will not strengthen his communicative behaviors.

GENERALIZED REINFORCERS. A generalized reinforcer is one that can be used to strengthen many different kinds of behaviors. One of the most common generalized reinforcers in our society is money. Others are praise, attention, affection, smiles, eye contact, and recognition. In order for a reinforcer to become a generalized reinforcer, it has to have been paired with a wide variety of primary or previously conditioned reinforcers (Hall, 1975; Hall & Fox, 1978). Money, for example, would not be a generalized reinforcer for an individual who had been institutionalized all of his life and had never had any experience with money. Nor would praise, attention, affection, smiles, eye contact, or recognition be generalized reinforcers for individuals who had spent their lives in situations which deprived them of these experiences. It is not uncommon for moderately to severely handicapped individuals to fail to respond to such common generalized reinforcers as we expect because they have not had enough, if any, experience with them.

However, generalized reinforcers are so desirable that it is particularly important to systematically pair them with primary and previously conditioned reinforcers so that they, too, become conditioned reinforcers — conditioned reinforcers that will reinforce a wide range of behaviors and also be readily available outside of structured situations.

INSTRUCTOR AS REINFORCER. One of the best criteria we know to determine whether an instructor is a superior instructor is to determine whether her approval or disapproval makes a difference to her students' behavior. Ideally, the instructor will establish herself as a positive reinforcer for students by initially taking some time to get acquainted, varying the amount and/or the kind of social and tangible consequences and responding appropriately and immediately to students' communicative attempts. This latter is most important because it keeps reinforcement within the context of the natural environment. For example, if a student says, "Wawa," "Want wawa," or "I want a glass of water, please," immediately give her a glass of water. In other words, reinforce a student whenever you have an opportunity to present a natural reinforcer that is appropriate to her communication.

In some cases, it is more difficult to establish yourself as a positive reinforcer for a student. When this occurs, it is necessary to pair your social praise and/or physical contact with previously established tangible reinforcers, such as tokens or primary reinforcers. Gradually reduce the amount of fruit, juice, tokens, or whatever tangible reinforcer you are using until they are no longer necessary, because the social consequences alone are effectively reinforcing the desired responses. Furthermore, you have become a discriminative stimulus for appropriate responding.

MICROSWITCHES. This section is included because microswitch designs allow many severely physically handicapped individuals to participate in home, school, and community activities that were previously denied to them. A microswitch can be arranged so that a severely physically handicapped student can activate it by raising her head or barely moving her finger, thus allowing this expressively communicatively impaired student to let us know a lot more about what she understands. Because microswitches respond immediately to a student's efforts, they can be extremely reinforcing.

The switches can reinforce students by signaling attention to them or by activating automated toys or games. They can also activate a variety of communicative devices, some of which will be discussed in Chapter 8. There are paddle switches which can be activated by hand pressure on top of the paddle. There are switches that can be activated by slight pressure on a vertical or horizontal flexible strip. There are switches that can be activated by pulling, grasping, or pinching. Combinations of these switches are also available (Wacker, 1983).

Summary

Select reinforcers that are currently being used in the home, classroom, or community settings with a student. Usually, this information could have been gleaned from preprogram observations. If an effective reinforcer has not already been established, it is essential to very reinforcers while keeping careful data in order to establish a reinforcer. The data recording sheets in Figure 4-1 may be used for this purpose. You may wish to review "Selecting Reinforcers" in Chapter 2 to refresh your memory on how to determine effective reinforcers.

What, When, and How to Reinforce

What to Reinforce

Generally, reinforce attending and all other appropriate behaviors exhibited by students. Certainly reinforce students for responding appropriately or attempting to respond appropriately to the discriminative stimuli you present. In addition to attending, which will be discussed in considerable detail in this chapter, the following communicative behaviors should be maintained or strengthened through reinforcement.

EYE CONTACT. Eye contact is one of the most common communicative techniques used by the nonhandicapped population to gain another person's attention or to express attending to another person. Eye contact is commonly a prerequisite communicative behavior to initiating a conversation. Frequently, moderately to severely handicapped individuals do not make eye contact. In fact, failure to make eye contact is often cited as one of the common characteristics of the autistic population. When you are instructing students who do not readily make eye contact, you must reinforce them when they do so in order to strenghten that natural, communicative behavior, in addition to providing appropriate discriminative stimuli for doing so in the form of instructing, modeling, prompting, and fading procedures.

BODY ORIENTATION. Body orientation is another common communicative technique used by the nonhandicapped population to express attending to another person. Again, moderately to severely handicapped individuals frequently do not exhibit this communicative behavior appropriately. Reinforce these individuals for facing you or others when they interact. Reinforce them for turning toward a new person who enters into a situation, thus recognizing and tacitly greeting the individual. Reinforce them for leaning toward those they interact with, rather than leaning back or to the side or turning away.

BODY POSITION. According to our definition, body position differs from body orientation in that, usually, it is only necessary to reinforce body position with those students who have moderate to severe physical as well as communicative handicaps. These students need to be reinforced for holding their heads upright, rather than resting their chins on their chests; for sitting or standing straight, rather than slumped over or slouching. Many of these students may always need braces and other prosthetic devices to support them. However, do not assume that all of the difficulties related to body positioning are the result of physical problems. Many of them are learned behaviors that are maintained or strengthened because they are reinforced. Consequently, reinforce normal or closer to normal body positions whenever they are exhibited. Not only are they communicative in and of themselves, but it is also obvious that a student would have considerable difficulty readily exhibiting communicative eye contact or body orientation unless the body were in an appropriate position to do so.

FACIAL EXPRESSIONS. Facial expressions often communicate more than one intends. This is true of both handicapped and nonhandicapped populations. If a student is explaining that it is impossible to respond appropriately in the communication and language session because of a tragedy at home and grinning all the while, the words lose their credibility. This visual and auditory incongruity may be present to an even greater extent with handicapped than nonhandicapped populations. Some of the specific facial expressions that should receive reinforcers are smiling as a greeting, raising eyes and eyebrows as a greeting or to express interest or pleasure *or* to communicate some question about what is going on, frowning to express disapproval or displeasure, and frowning or grimacing to express fear.

COMMUNICATIVE GESTURES. There are so many obvious and subtle communicative gestures that an entire chapter easily could be devoted to them. In fact, Mehrabian (1972) claims that only 7 percent of what we communicate to others is actually communicated by the words we select and that of the remaining 93 percent, 55 percent is communicated by body language, including gestures. This is for normal speakers. In our experience, many individuals who have difficulty speaking seem to use more gestures, facial expressions, postures, etc., to express themselves than the average person does, so it is certainly worthwhile to teach them communicative gestures which, later, can be accompanied by speaking, signing, or other forms of symbolic communication.

Pointing, showing, giving, head nodding or shaking, and hand waving or shaking are all examples of communicative gestures (Bates, 1979). Reinforce students for pointing to something they want or that is of interest. Reinforce them for showing you something by handing it to you. Reinforce them for giving you something as a gift or as a way of communicating that they want you to interact with them and the object. Reinforce students for nodding their heads to indicate "yes" or shaking their heads to indicate "no." Reinforce clapping to express approval, waving "hello" or "goodbye" or to signal someone, placing a finger to the lips to indicate "be quiet," motioning with finger or entire hand or arm for someone to approach, raising hand or hand and forearm for someone to stay away, shaking hands to greet someone, patting or hugging to express approval or pleasure, tilting head to one side to express some question, and shrugging shoulders to express failure to understand.

IMITATING MOTOR RESPONSES. Some moderately to severely communicatively impaired students may not have learned how to imitate simple motor responses. When this is the case, motor imitation must be taught in order for students to learn to use communicative gestures. These students should be reinforced for imitating clapping, waving, and other communicative motor responses, or for making responses that are steps in the direction of imitating these motor behaviors (Murdock & Hartmann, 1975). These are communicative gestures with which most students can experience some success. Not only is it important to start a student at a level where he can experience a lot of success, but, as noted in Chapter 2 and on the checklist and spontaneous communication and language sample records, gestures, facial expressions, etc., are critical components of the total process.

RECEPTIVE LANGUAGE. In teaching phonology, morphology and syntax, the emphasis in this program is on *expressive* language. This is not because we see receptive language as being less important than language production, but rather because receiving and processing language is often more obscure than production and production is easier to observe and record. It is sometimes very difficult to determine just how much an individual comprehends. Furthermore, receptive language is often learned while mastering production (Gray & Ryan, 1973).

Nevertheless, you want to reinforce indications of receptive language as much as possible. A student can be reinforced whenever she responds appropriately to what is said, for example, when she follows directions or instructions; or when she points or otherwise identifies particular nouns, verbs, adjectives, etc. In some instances, the student will already have much of this receptive language when you begin instructing her, thus providing frequent opportunities for you to reinforce her socially for her communicative skills. Intersperse receptive language tasks between trials on new, more difficult expressive language tasks. When you do this, give her whatever reinforcer you would have given her for succeeding on the more difficult expressive task.

CONVERSATIONAL TURN-TAKING. Reinforce conversational turn-taking. Many communicatively impaired individuals fail to develop interactional skills when talking to others. They often respond only to certain questions or specific requests to say something. Their conversational skills are poor and they fail to use spontaneously and naturally the communication and language skills they have acquired.

People in the students' environments can be trained to teach them how to use the basics of conversational turn-taking (MacDonald, 1982). Communicatively impaired individuals can be encouraged to take these turns by (1) involving them in activities that interest them, (2) presenting them with models they can match in length and syntactic and morphological complexity, (3) waiting for them to respond to their conversational partner, and (4) signaling them nonverbally and, if need be, verbally if they fail to take their turn. MacDonald suggests that turn-taking with gestures and actions with objects can lead into vocal and then verbal conversational turn-taking.

In CLIP, conversational turns are incorporated in step 3 of Table 3-2, the sample teaching format for syntactic and morphological structures. In this step, the instructor presents one or two models of the target structure appropriate to the student's current activity, then he waits with obvious expectancy for the student to take her turn and respond. If she doesn't respond within 5 to 10 seconds, the instructor signals by a gesture to take a turn or makes a verbal request for a response (e.g., "Your turn," "What do you say?" etc.). If the student doesn't respond, a model or a partial model may need to be presented again. Nonverbal and verbal prompts that a turn is expected from the student should eventually be faded until just eye contact, waiting, or other behaviors that naturally occur in normal conversational environments signal the student that it is her turn. Waiting for the student to respond, and then responding in return, often serve as natural reinforcers for conversational turn-taking.

EXPRESSIVE LANGUAGE. Reinforce correct communication and language responses and approximations to correct responses, including phonology, syntax, and morphology. Reinforce a student for responding correctly whether he responds with a communicative gesture or with a spoken seven-word sentence. Considering a previous example, if you and a student have been eating salted popcorn and you say, "I'm thirsty. I want a glass of water. What do you want?" and the student responds, "I want a glass of water," immediately praise him and give him the water as a reinforcer because this is a natural response to the question. However, since there was no instruction involved in the request from you which would indicate to the student that he was to respond in a complete sentence, you would give him the water and praise him if he had simply responded, "Water" or "Wawa," depending upon his communicative skills. Furthermore, you would reinforce another student for raising his hand to his lips as though he were holding a glass. See the previous section on "Establishing

Specific Language Structures" for more details regarding syntactic, morphological, and phonological structures that should be reinforced.

PROSODY. While Mehrabian (1972) attributed only 7 percent of the communication process to the actual words the speaker selects and 55 percent to body language, the remaining 38 percent is related to prosody. Prosody simply means the rhythmic patterns and modulation of the voice. For example, many times we don't actually hear the words, but we pick up on the speaking patterns and we understand. Consider also how a sarcastic tone of voice reverses the meaning of the words or how an upward inflection pattern at the end of the sentence turns a statement into a question.

Reinforce the student socially and, when necessary, with tangible reinforcers for using appropriate intonation, pitch, stress, and duration patterns. Be sure your vocal patterns model natural prosody. Avoid models such as "The (pause) girl (pause) is (pause) running," where each word slides around at least three different tones and the statement is delivered so slowly that the listener has forgotten the beginning by the time the speaker gets to the end. Also, avoid stereotypic models or ones with target structures overemphasized when such overemphasis is no longer necessary. For example, "Daddy *is* home" when "Daddy's home" would be more natural.

Frequently, it helps to use tactile and/or kinesthetic stimuli to prompt appropriate prosody. Take the student's hand or arm and move it in rhythm with what you are trying to teach her to say as you say it. If necessary, use this tactile and kinesthetic prompt as you get her to say it with you. Such unison talking paired rhythmic physical movement is a very strong but very useful prompting procedure.

SUCCESSIVE APPROXIMATIONS TO TARGET BEHAVIORS. Whenever you are shaping behaviors, reinforce a successive approximation to the target behavior, that is, something that is close to the final response you are working toward or at least something that is a step in the right direction. If the student cannot follow simple instructions or make the correct response by imitating you or after having been given the strongest prompt in the teaching format, you can shape his behavior by reinforcing the closest approximation to the correct response that he can make. For example, if you are trying to get him to say "water," reinforce only those sounds which more closely resemble the word "water," such as "wawa." As a consequence, the student's speech sounds will shift in the direction of the word that you are trying to teach him (Sloane, Johnston, & Harris, 1968). Gradually change your criterion for the sounds you will reinforce, requiring closer and closer approximations to the correct production of the word "water."

Once again, we cannot overemphasize the importance of a high success rate for these students. Thus, it is often necessary to use shaping procedures. They must be provided with an opportunity to do many things right so that they can receive reinforcers that they have earned. This is vital not only to how well they will attend and work in the communication and language instructional sessions but also to their developing more positive self-concepts.

When to Reinforce

Normally, reinforce the student immediately after he makes a correct response. There should be minimal delay between the time the student responds correctly and when he receives his reinforcer. This is to eliminate the possibility of another behavior occurring between the correct response and the reinforcer, particularly an undesirable behavior such as gazing off into space, hands-in-mouth, or grabbing teaching materials. It is importnt to understand that a reinforcer will strenghten any response it follows. Consequently, care must be taken not to reinforce or strengthen undesirable behaviors. If optimal learning is to occur, reinforcers must be delivered only contingent upon correct responding. Optimal learning for the purposes of communication and language tasks is defined as requiring successively fewer trials to mastery of new tasks and responding correctly at 80 percent or better (Alberto & Troutman, 1982; Axelrod, 1983; Becker et al., 1971; Hall, 1975; Hall & Fox, 1978; Murdock, 1978a; Sloane & MacAulay, 1968).

How to Reinforce

Use natural reinforcers whenever possible. For example, give the student things she asks for whenever it is reasonable to do so. Respond socially to social communication from her. Listen to her when she tries to communicate.

Reinforce a student by simply presenting social consequences for appropriate behaviors whenever it is possible. Praise her, smile at her, pat her on the shoulder, shake her hand, or provide any combination of social reinforcers. If you are also using tangible or activity reinforcers, social reinforcers must be paired with whatever tangible or activity reinforcer you have determined is necessary.

Reinforcers should not interfere with ongoing instruction. Just as it is wiser to use tangible primary reinforcers that can be consumed as readily as a squirt of fruit juice, it may also be wiser to give check marks or plus marks than poker chips or other tokens that the student might drop, rattle, or play with instead of attending to you. There are many activity reinforcers that are natural in home, school, and community settings. These activities should be arranged so that an activity a student desires less precedes one that is more desirable; thus, the more desirable activity reinforces the less desirable activity (Premack, 1959). For example, if Elizabeth freely engages in going to the yard to swing and does so whenever she has the opportunity, but matches and folds the recently laundered socks only when there's a payoff, let her fold socks first, then swing.

Other effective ways to deliver reinforcers include presenting a choice and variety of reinforcers at unpredictable times. A surprise is usually very reinforcing and also very effective as far as developng persistence. If a student knows exactly what she is working for, she may decide that the completion of the task is not worth the effort involved. If the specific reinforcement possibilities are unknown, she may very well work longer and with more interest for what is really a surprise reward (Hall & Fox, 1978).

In the final analysis, how you reinforce a student depends upon the unique characteristics of that student. There may be students for whom only things that take as long to chew as a caramel or are as concrete as a poker chip are reinforcing. When this is the case, initially you give them the caramel or the poker chip, but you pair such consequences with things that are less distracting until these neutral or nonreinforcing stimuli are conditioned to take on the same reinforcing properties as the caramels or the poker chips. There may also be individuals who do not respond well to surprises but who respond optimally in an extremely routine, predictable environment. There may even be individuals whom you cannot praise, hug, pat, or smile at initially because these are not reinforcing events for them. Again, you must pair these social consequences with whatever is reinforcing until they, too, become conditioned reinforcers. It's easy to say, "Reinforcers strengthen behaviors, therefore, give a person a reinforcer for any behavior you want to strengthen." However, it's not always easy to determine precisely what that reinforcer is.

Reinforcement Schedules

Reinforcers can be delivered on ratio or interval schedules. A ratio schedule depends upon the number of responses and an interval schedule depends upon the passage of time between responses (Alberto & Troutman, 1982; Axelrod, 1983; Hall, 1975; Hall & Fox, 1978; Murdock, 1978a; Sloane, Buckholdt, Jensen, & Crandall, 1979).

Only ratio schedules will be discussed in detail here because CLIP's sample teaching format and data recording sheet lend themselves well to collecting ratio data which, in this instance, is simply trial-by-trial data. Furthermore, the recording and graphing procedures described in Chapter 4 are much more suited to ratio data collection. Continuous, fixed, and variable ratio reinforcement schedules will be discussed, emphasizing the effect the latter has upon persistence.

CONTINUOUS REINFORCEMENT SCHEDULE. Continuous reinforcement (CRF) involves reinforcing every correct response. When delivering tangible reinforcers, they should be delivered after every correct response or on a CRF schedule when the student is learning a new task. Continuous reinforcement is also the most effective schedule to use when shaping behavior (Hall, 1975). Whenever you give a student a tangible reiforcer, pair it with a social reinforcer. As soon as a student demonstrates mastery of a particular task by reaching criteria, move to the following fixed-ratio reinforcement schedule.

FIXED—RATIO REINFORCEMENT SCHEDULES. A fixed-ratio reinforcement schedule simply means that a fixed number of correct responses is reinforced (Alberto & Troutman, 1982; Axelrod, 1983; Hall, 1975; Hall & Fox, 1978, Murdock, 1978a). This could be every second, third, fourth, or hundredth correct response. After a student has mastered a task to whatever criteria you have established, we recommend thinning the tangible reinforcers by reinforcing every other correct response until he is reliably responding on this reiforcement schedule. This is known as a fixed ratio of two or FR 2 reinforcement schedule. You must be very careful not to remain on a fixed-ratio reinforcement schedule because behaviors maintained on these schedules can extinguish very quickly when the student is no longer receiving reinforcers.

Making Communication and Language Behaviors Persistent

VARIABLE—RATIO REINFORCEMENT SCHEDULES. In order to establish persistent communication and language behaviors, behaviors that are highly resistant to extinction, continue to thin the reinforcement schedule for tangibles to what is referred to as a variable-ratio reinforcement schedule. A variable-ratio reinforcement schedule is simply one in which a variable number of correct responses is reinforced (Alberto & Troutman, 1982; Axelrod, 1983; Hall, 1975; Hall & Fox, 1978; Murdock, 1978a). When correct responding is consistent on the FR 2 schedule, we recommend moving to a variable ratio of reinforcing about every third correct response or a VR 3 ratio. Out of 10 correct responses, the student would be reinforced about three times, making sure that reinforcers are not delivered on exactly every third correct response but on an unpredictable, intermittent schedule. It is the unpredictability that makes behaviors persistent. Even with moderately to severely handicapped students, plan on thinning the reinforcers to about a VR 5 schedule. Table 3-2, the teaching format for syntactic and morphological structures, provides an example of how to list these reinforcement schedules sequentially, from the beginning to the end of training (cf. Murdock & Hartman, 1975).

As a student reaches criteria on one reinforcement schedule, move sequentially through the remaining schedules until you eventually reach at least a VR 5 reinforcement schedule. Do not hesitate to explore the effectiveness of an even thinner variable-ratio reinforcement schedule. The more unpredictable the reinforcer delivery is, the more persistent the behavior is. The following is a summary of the foregoing recommended reinforcement schedules:

CRF: Reinforce every correct response.
FR 2: Reinforce every other correct response.
VR 3: Reinforce about every third correct response.
VR 5: Reinforce about every fifth correct response.

Social reinforcers or consequences that are natural to an utterance or a communicative attempt can always be delivered on a continuous reinforcement schedule, particularly when doing so is appropriate to the situation. For example, every time a student communicates appropriately, respond naturally to him by answering his questions, giving him what he asks for, or engaging in a conversation. Also praise him, smile at him, hug him, recognize his accomplishment with your eye contact, or otherwise reinforce him socially.

GUIDELINES FOR STRUCTURING A COMMUNICATION AND LANGUAGE SESSION

For most speech-language pathologists or special education teachers, normally there will be one or more designated periods during a school day which are scheduled as "communication training" and/or "language instruction." This section provides specific teaching suggestions related to these more structured instructional settings.

Trials

Quite simply, a trial consists of the following: The instructor presents (1) verbal and (2) visual stimuli and (3) a prompt if necessary. Then (4) the student responds and (5) the instructor reinforcers a correct response either socially or socially and tangibly or, in the event the response is incorrect, the instructor repeats the task, providing the prompt required to get a correct response. These numbers correspond to those across the top of the teaching format and the data recording sheet.

NUMBER OF TRIALS IN A SESSION. The number of trials in any one session may vary considerably depending upon the attending level of the student, the number of tasks you are attempting to cover in that session, and the difficulty of the material. It is important that the student experience a high level of success, at least a 70 to 80 percent success level during each session.

Consequently, if new material is very difficult, intersperse it generously with review tasks so that the student can succeed and be reinforced. If the student is still not responding with 70 to 80 percent, (1) provide a stronger prompt, (2) vary or increase the reinforcers, or (3) move to a simpler task.

Normally, plan on presenting a minimum of ten trials for a total of three to five new tasks. This will give a minimum of 30 to 50 trials on new material per session and allow for extensive review of previously mastered material. The exception to this would be a student who masterd the new material very quickly. When a student gets five unprompted consecutive trials correct, it is not necessary to continue repeating the task in order to record ten trials. Simply assume that subsequent trials would be correct and give the student credit for them. Normally, plan on presenting at least 10 to 20 trials on any particular task that you are trying to teach a student.

Scoring spaces for a maximum of 20 trials on any given task are included on the data recording sheet since you may decide that for the particular student you are working with, a minimum of 20 trials on each new task is desirable. This decision would be based on his attending level, the necessity for repetition, and how much review is involved. While selecting a minimum of 20 trials would double the above figure, there should be ample time to complete a session in 20 to 30 minutes.

After a student has mastered a task, make certain that discriminative stimuli are varied. For instance, if you are trying to teach her to say "mama," you might ask her "Who is this?" (when her mother is present), or "Who brought you to school today?" (when you know her mother brought her), or present her with a visual stimulus, such as a picture of her mother, and ask her "Who is this?" Thus, you are presenting a variety of discriminative stimuli that all require the same response.

Movement From Task to Task Within a Session

Do not repeat the same task for 10 consecutive trials during the session, particularly if the student is not experiencing a lot of success on the task, but rather move to another task whenever the student has (1) either responded correctly without prompts for three trials or (2) responded correctly after being prompted followed by at least two unprompted correct responses. In other words, when a student makes an error, at least three or four trials are presented on that particular task. This is important in order to stabilize the correct response. Too often instructors tend to move on to another task as soon as a student responds correctly, thus missing the ideal opportunity to begin to stabilize that behavior. Very few nonhandicapped individuals have mastered a new behavior just because they are able to get it right once. This is particularly so for moderately to severely communicatively impaired individuals.

If a student does not respond correctly after the second prompt, discontinue working on that task and immediately interject several review tasks which the student has mastered well so that he can be reinforced for responding correctly and experience some success. Then return to the task he failed, making certain that a stronger prompt is provided. If he still cannot respond correctly, provide more review items so that he can once again experience some success. If the student cannot respond correctly on the task he failed when you have provided the strongest prompt at least twice, move to an easier task that will give him more success experiences and, possibly, prerequisite skills that he needs to perform successfully on the task he has been failing.

Session Length

A session may last up to 30 minutes, depending upon the attending level of the student. It has been our experience that after the teaching routine has become established, even severely impaired or multiply handicapped students can attend and cooperate for up to 20 or 30 minutes if the session moves rapidly and the instructor is enthusiastic and reinforcing.

ESTABLISHING ATTENDING BEHAVIORS

Attending is essential to learning. A student cannot learn a task when she does not attend to its model or her own execution of it. Attending is often defined as having the student look at the instructor or other appropriate visual stimuli for three seconds or more following attention signals from the instructor (Murdock & Hartmann, 1975). You have not yet asked the student to do anything except watch you and listen. However, the ultimate criterion for attending is whether the student attempts to respond in a manner that is appropriate to the task's instructions. For example, if you and the student are eating lunch and you show her the eating utensils and say, "Point to the spoon," and she does so, she is obviously attending to you and to your instructions. If she points to the fork, she has also demonstrated that she is attending in that she has tried to respond correctly, although she has made an error. When such an error occurs, you should provide her with a prompt that will help her to respond correctly, such as showing her the spoon. However, if the student simply points randomly at any object that happens to be available (e.g., a ring you happen to be wearing), she is *not* attending and attending must be established before you can proceed.

To establish attending behaviors, present verbal instructions simply and clearly by saying, "Angela, watch me. Listen" (Murdock & Hartmann, 1975). This watch-me-listen signal should be paired with the student's name and with a visual signal also, gesturing with your hand by first holding it next to your face at eye level as you say, "Watch me," and then moving your hand back toward your ear as you say "Listen." Such gesturing is effective because it not only adds additional communication cues, but later on the gestures alone or just saying the student's name will often serve as reminders or signals for the watch and listen (Axelrod, 1983, Becker et al., 1971; Hall, 1975; Sloane et al., 1979).

Do not distract the student with the reinforcer. Whenever you are using a tangible reinforcer, hold it near your face, the object, the picture, or whatever it may be that you want the student to visually attend to. Holding a reinforcer off to the side is almost guaranteeing that the student will not attend to the communication or language task that you are presenting because the reinforcer is distracting her.

You might reinforce another student for attending so that nonattending students like Angela can see that attending pays off. Use descriptive praise. For example, say, "Very good, Sam. I like the way you're getting ready to work." If Angela fails to imitate Sam's model, model the appropriate behavior for her yourself by saying, "Very good sitting still and watching, Ms. Abercrombie!" as you give yourself a reinforcer (Murdock & Hartmann, 1975).

If none of the above succeed, physically prompt her by placing her in the correct attending posture. Then reinforce her for attending. Use descriptive praise and other social reinforcers, as well as any tangible reinforcer that you may be using.

Caution should be used here to ensure that you are not inadvertently reinforcing nonattending behaviors by talking to or physically touching the student when she is not attending (Murdock & Hartmann, 1975). The only way you can be sure of this is by keeping accurate data to determine whether attending behavior is increasing (Murdock & Hartmann, 1975). If it is not, something is maintaining or strengthening the nonattending behaviors and, possibly, it's something you're doing. Therefore, implement the followng time-out procedure:

1. Turn your head away and totally withdraw your attention and materials from the student. Do not respond to her until she has stopped her nonattending activities for about three seconds to a full minute (Murdock & Hartmann, 1975). The object is to make certain that you are not inadvertently reinforcing a student's nonattending behaviors. Sometimes it is very difficult to determine what is maintaining or strengthening nonattending behaviors. It could be something as subtle as your eye contact. Therefore, it becomes necessary for you not to even look at the student.
2. Reinforce attending. As soon as the student has ceased her nonattending activities for about three seconds and appears ready to attend, turn and face her squarely, smile at her, reinforce her for attending, and present the communication or language task on which you are working.

ELIMINATING INTERFERING BEHAVIORS

Moderately to severely communicatively impaired students may exhibit many behaviors that interfere with your teaching and their learning. Some have stereotyped behaviors such as rocking back and forth, shaking their heads, flipping their hands or fingers, etc. Others put their hands in their mouths or over their eyes. Others grab at you and/or your teaching materials. All of these are examples of behaviors that must be eliminated because they interfere with a student's ability to attend appropriately and learn.

Establish Appropriate Incompatible Behaviors

If a student exhibits hand-in-mouth, hands-over-eyes, or grabbing behaviors, etc., establish hands-in-pockets, arm-folding, or hands-in-lap behaviors (Murdock & Hartmann, 1975). You may be able to establishing appropriate behaviors by modeling them yourself or using another student as a model. Ignore interfering behaviors while simultaneously reinforcing any appropriate behavior that the student exhibits, particularly one that is incompatible with the interfering behavior. Reinforcing appropriate incompatible behaviors is an excellent procedure to use to weaken or eliminate inappropriate behaviors (Axelrod, 1983; Becker et al., 1971; Hall, 1975; Murdock, 1978a; Sloane et al., 1979). It is not possible for a student to have his hands in his lap or his arms folded and at the same time have them over his eyes, in this mouth or grabbing instructional materials.

This procedure is applicable to many problem behaviors. An individual cannot be flipping his hands or his fingers or twirling his hair if his hands or arms are folded. Whenever you can reinforce or strengthen a desirable behavior that is incompatible with an undesirable behavior, do so. This creates a much more positive and effective instructional environment than one that centers around scolding or otherwise punishing students.

It may be necessary to prompt the student by physically moving him through the arm-folding or hands-in-lap or any other incompatible, appropriate behaviors. Gradually fade out this physical prompting and reinforce the student each time he gets closer to the desired response (Murdock & Hartmann, 1975; Sloane et al., 1979).

Increase or Vary Reinforcers

If undesirable behaviors continue, it may be that the reward you are presenting for desirable responses is not, in fact, reinforcing or, if it is reinforcing, you may not be giving him enough of it. Consequently, you should explore increasing the amount of the reinforcer first and, if that fails, vary the rewards until you find an effective reinforcer.

Implement a Time-Out Procedure

Paying attention to the interfering behaviors may be responsible for maintaining or even strengthening them (Axelrod, 1983; Becker et al, 1971; Hall, 1975; Murdock & Hartmann, 1975). In some cases, it may be necessary to remove your attention *completely* from the student by turning away, putting your head down and to the side, and withdrawing all attention from the student as described in the section on "Attending." (With students who grab, throw, or shove things, it may be necessary to remove materials also.) This is a mild form of time-out. If this fails, try a stronger time-out procedure by placing the student in an isolated area for as short a period of time as possible but for as long it takes for his interfering behaviors to cease. As soon as they cease, promptly return him to the teaching setting, without commenting on his interfering behaviors, and present him with the attention watch-me-listen signal and the communication or langauge task as quickly as possible before he can start his interfering behaviors again (Axelrod, 1983; Becker et al, 1971; Hall, 1975; Murdock, 1978a; Sloane et al., 1979).

Present a Mild Punishment Procedure

LOUD NOISE. If all of the above fail and a student continues to emit a high rate of a specific inappropriate behavior, it may be necessary to present an aversive stimulus immediately following that inappropriate behavior. For example, you might loudly verbalize, "No!" paired with a sharp rap on the table or desk or with a lound handclap (Murdock & Hartmann, 1975). This mild punishment procedure has a startle effect on the student which almost inevitably results in his stopping the undesirable behavior. When this happens, immediately present him with a task that is relevant to the ongoing teaching and praise him and otherwise reinforce him generously both for attending and for responding appropriately.

PHYSICAL RESTRAINT. With some students it may be necessary to physically restrain them in order to get them to stop engaging in interfering behaviors and to attend to you. A mild form of physical restraint is to seat the student and hold him in the chair by placing your hands on his shoulders, without commenting. When more restraint is necessary, sit with the student facing you and place his knees between yours and his hands between his knees. Your hands are free to hold his head if necessary so that he is facing you. Obviously such restraint is not pleasant, but it is possible that it seems more unpleasant to you than it actually is for the student. However, his hands are not free to use gestures or to point. Consequently, reinforce him generously for eye contact or other signs of attending and gradually remove such forms of restraint, beginning with releasing his head, then one hand at a time, then not holding his knees quite so securely, etc., as you reinforce him for sitting and keeping his hands or arms folded.

Summary of Ways to Eliminate Interfering Behaviors

In summary, ultimately, interfering behaviors must be eliminated. Ideally, inappropriate behaviors are eliminated by strengthening or establishing behaviors that are incompatible with them. In order to do this, first try requesting and/or modeling the desirable behavior and then reinforcing the student's appropriate reponse. If that fails, go through each of the following procedures in sequence until you find one that is effective:

1. Check to make certain that you have a reinforcer.
2. Reinforce all appropriate responses, particularly those that are incompatible with interfering behaviors.
3. Ignore inappropriate behaviors while simulataneously reinforcing appro-

priate behaviors.
4. Prompt the student to respond appropriately by physically moving her through the correct response.
5. Increase or vary reinforcers.
6. Use a time-out procedure.
7. Present a mild punishment procedure.
8. Physically restrain the student.

SUMMARY OF TEACHING PROCEDURES

Communication and language intervention for moderately to severely communicatively impaired students belongs in the natural environment and, insofar as possible, using materials which are natural also. These students need to be presented with many opportunities to practice their recently acquired communicative skills and to learn new skills throughout their waking hours. Adults and others who interact with them should be responsive to their spontaneous communicative attempts and understand instructional procedures well enough to utilize and, when necessary, arrange natural environments so that an abundance of cues and consequences will be available. This is essential both for initial acquisition and for appropriate generalization.

In order to acquire communication and language behaviors, moderately to severely communicatively impaired populations must learn to discriminate stimuli that signal or cue communicative responses. These responses can be established through instructing, modeling, prompting, shaping, and/or chaining procedures. Once communication and language behaviors are established, they are maintained and/or strengthened through reinforcement. There are many types of reinforcers. Instructors have to vary these in both kind and amount until students are responding optimally, with optimal responding determined by fewer trials to criterion as well as a high rate of correct responding. Natural reinforcers are very desirable because they are much more likely to be used by others with whom students come into contact and they are also more likely to be generalized reinforcers.

The most important consideration regarding selecting reinforcers, however, is the effect they have on the student's responding. Therefore, use whatever reinforcer is necessary, including primary reinforcers or tokens, to reduce the time it takes to master new behaviors and to increase the rate of correct responding once communicative behaviors are established. However, primary or token reinforcers must be paired with other more naturally occurring stimuli so that the naturally occurring stimuli will take on the same reinforcing properties as edibles or tokens.

Reinforce *all* appropriate communicative behaviors and attempts to communicate immediately with social reinforces. Thin tangible reinforcer delivery to an unpredictable, intermittent reinforcement schedule in order to make communication and language behaviors persistent.

Attending behaviors must be established and interfering behaviors eliminated in order for students to learn. However, these are not to be thought of as separate goals to be accomplished before actual communication and language instruction can begin. Attending *is* a communicative behavior and it is one of the first that both handicapped and nonhandicapped individuals need to learn. Increasing attending and other appropriate behaviors is one of the most effective ways to decrease or eliminate interfering behaviors.

CHAPTER 4

RECORDING AND GRAPHING DATA: ACCOUNTABILITY

JANE Y. MURDOCK

ANY systematic method of making observations will provide information about what is being learned. Simply keeping daily data and graphing it can show you *what* the individual you are teaching is learning as well as how *fast* she is learning it. However, these data do not make it possible to assume that it was *your* teaching that caused the learning to occur.

This section will provide you with procedures to determine the cause-effect relationship between your teaching and communicatively impaired individuals' learning. In other words, you can be accountable for your instruction. Keeping accurate records of each communicatively handicapped individual's performance and responding to those data are essential to the success of this program. Your data determine the following aspects of your treatment procedures:

1. The particular communicative task that you select to teach.
2. Whether you prompt and what prompting procedure you use.
3. The reinforcement schedule you should use.
4. Whether it is necessary to use shaping procedures.
5. When you change from task to task within a session.
6. When a task becomes a review task.
7. When to move to a new task.

Consequently, it is fundamental to the success of this program that you not only record your data accurately initially but that you also put it in a form that readily reflects performance. This chapter describes how to record and graph these data. It concludes with a discussion of accountability and recommends procedures that can be used in the classroom, home, and community that will assure you and others of the effectiveness of your communication and language intervention procedures. These are designed so as to minimize disrupting normal activities in these environments.

RECORDING PROCEDURES

Data should be recorded immediately following each trial. Use the data recording sheet in Figure 4-1 for this purpose. The type of recording to be used is trial-by-trial recording. Each trial is recorded using the following code based on the response: correct (+), incorrect (−), prompted correct (p+), prompted incorrect (p−), or no response(0). You may choose not to use the prompted or no-response codes but rather simply to record those as incorrect responses. I recommend using them because of the additional information they provide regarding the individual's performance in each particular language session. Recorded responses are defined as follows:

1. *A correct response* (+) is recorded whenever the response to the presented stimuli is correct without being prompted.
2. *An incorrect response* (−) is recorded whenever any response is made other than the defined correct response for the presented stimuli.
3. *A prompted correct response* (p+) is recorded whenever the response is correct after having been prompted by the instructor.
4. *A prompted incorrect response* (p−) is recorded whenever any response is made other than the correct response after having been prompted by the instructor.
5. *No response* (0) is recorded whenever there is no response made to the presented stimuli within five seconds.

Count the number of *correct (+) responses only* and divide this total by the total number of trials on a particular task in a given session. Multiply this figure by 100 to find the percentage correct on a given task. For example, if 10 trials on a particular task were presented and the individual you were instructing got 4 correct (+), 2 incorrect (−) and 4 prompted correct (p+), you would divide the 4 correct responses by 10, the total number of trials, giving you 0.4. You multiply 0.4 by 100 in order to change the decimal into a percentage score. Thus, your student would have 40 percent on that particular task (Murdock & Hartmann, 1975).

GRAPHING DATA

Graph the percentage correct for each task immediately if possible but at least daily in order to facilitate planning for the next session's task selection, reinforcement schedule, and prompting procedures. A graph gives you a clear visual representation of the data. Individuals with severe communication and language disorders may not seem to be making very much progress; thus, instructors tend to become discouraged unless they have some evidence that what they are doing is, in fact, working. On the other hand, a graph provides you with the feedback you need in order to change reinforcers, prompts, and/or tasks when a student's progress is not adequate.

Figure 4-1

DATA RECORDING SHEET*

Student________________ Instructor________________ General Objectives: VIRSDRCC

Date	Discriminative Stimuli (Instructor)			Response (Student)	Consequent Stimuli (Instructor)	Correct (+) Incorrect (-) Prompted Correct (p+) Prompted Incorrect (p-) No Response (0)	%** Correct
	Verbal	Visual	Prompt				

*Adapted from Murdock and Hartmann (1975). **Calculate only correct (+) responses.

Making It Simple

Graphing data can be as simple as recording data. Mark "Percentage Correct" on the vertical axis and write in 0 to 100 from bottom to top on the graph. Mark "Session Number" across the bottom of the graph on the horizontal axis. Put the name of the person you are instructing and the language task depicted on that graph at the top. You can use one graph for several tasks if you use a coding system to distinguish them. This is very simple if you use different colors to make the data points and connect the lines. Do not use colors if you anticipate making photocopies of your graphs but, rather, use symbols such as X's, O's, or circles, squares, triangles, etc., to distinguish the different tasks represented by each data point. Calculate the percentages correct and record them on the appropriate graph(s) after each communication training session.

Figure 4-2

EXAMPLE OF SIMPLE GRAPH DESIGNED TO DEPICT TWO COMMUNICATIVE TASKS

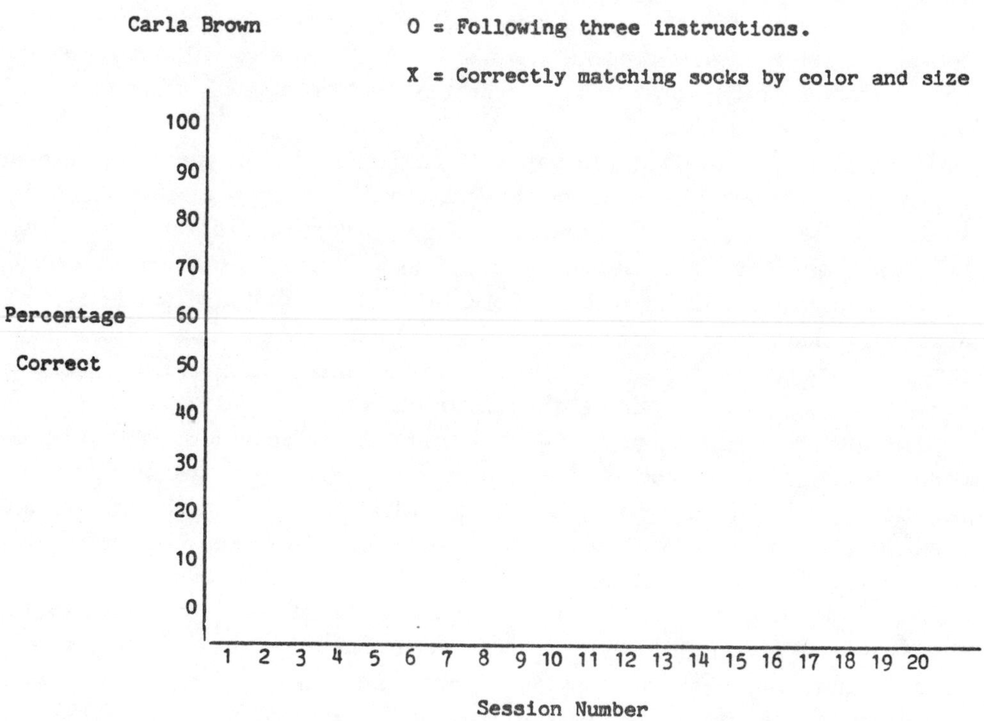

This graph will provide all of the information you need to see at a glance from the data you recorded whether the student requires stronger prompts or reinforcers or whether she has reached criterion on any of the tasks depicted. As a result of these data, you can fill in the date, appropriate tasks, reinforcers, reinforcement schedules, prompting procedures, and discriminative stimuli on the data recording sheet for the next session. It only takes a few minutes to keep accurate data and plan lessons if you follow these procedures.

ACCOUNTABILITY

Many speech-language pathologists, special educators and other professionals tend to feel threatened by the word *accountability.* This is particularly so when they are working with severely handicapped populations and the accountability is evaluated by administering one or more standardized communication or language tests before and after the intervention program. In order to demonstrate accountability under such circumstances, you have to prove statistically that the gains your students made were significant at some predetermined probability level, usually at least .05.

There are several problems with this, particularly when applied to a moderately to severely handicapped population. First, usually a control group is required. Consequently, approximately half of your moderately or severely communicatively impaired population conceivably could go without receiving any instruction until you had demonstrated the effectiveness of your procedures with the other half.

Second, there is an assumption that the control group and the group receiving the instruction can be compared to each other. In order to do this, for every student in the communication and language intervention program there must be another student who is not in the program who has the same communication and language abilities (or lack of abilities), as well as being matched on all other variables considered relevant, such as IQ, chronological age, mental age, sex, race, socioeconomic status, etc. This is extremely difficult, if not close to impossible, with such small and diverse populations.

The third problem has to do with individualizing instruction. In traditional group designs, data are collected on a number of individuals, preferably a large number, which we rarely have available with either moderately or severely handicapped populations. Then, overall scores are reported on the entire test and, when there are subtests, teachers and parents occasionally get these scores, also. However, it is the mean or average performance of each group that is determined, and individual data are lost in the process. Nevertheless, special educators, speech-language pathologists, and others working with handicapped students are required to write individualized education programs (IEP's) for every student in their charge.

Finally, testing administered for group designs typically provides only a small sample of communication skills taken at a given point in time. Single-subject designs provide ongoing, continuous assessment of each individual's communication skills and the progress he or she is making. Ongoing assessment alerts you to unsatisfactory progress so that you can alter your instructional strategies accordingly. It also provides you with clear evidence when communication gains are being made that they are the result of your efforts and not just fortuitous accidents.

I recommend using single-subject research designs which will provide not only teachers and speech-language pathologists with the individualized information they require but which are relatively simple techniques for parents and paraprofessionals to use also. I have found that the feedback provided by these procedures is extremely reinforcing for anyone engaging in communication and language intervention or other programs with moderately to severely handicapped populations where traditional, standardized testing may not indicate significant gains because an exceptional population is being compared to the mythical normal mean.

Single-subject designs will make it possible to monitor the performance of individuals and record it daily, or even more frequently, over an extended period of time. Each communicatively impaired individual is compared only to himself by inspecting his performance during the baseline (before your communication instruction) condition and then during the intervention (after you begin communication instruction) conditions. Consequently, each student serves as his own experimental control, which obviates the difficulties in group designs with small samples and random sampling.

Baseline Data

Baseline data are essential to any single-subject design. Baseline data simply reflect the level of the communication skills *before* you begin the communication and language intervention program. When you are collecting baseline data, you do not use the instructional procedures described in CLIP and, normally, the student does not receive any reinforcers or feedback, not even about how to correct mistakes. It is necessary to say "normally" because frequently there are instances where some reinforcing and/or other feedback are occurring when you enter into the situation. When this is the case, baseline data should be taken that reflect whatever happens to be going on immediately before you begin your communication and language instruction using CLIP. This is one of the hazards of taking data in home, school, or community environments as opposed to laboratory environments where arrangements can be made for virgin subjects, uncontaminated by previous treatment procedures.

Baseline data are actually similar to pretests in that they provide a measure of the communication and language behaviors (dependent variables) before your intervention procedures (independent variables). Normally, the baseline data recommended here provide a much larger sample of the targeted behaviors. Data are collected continuously both during baseline and after intervention. These two measurements can later be compared to see if noticeable differences are present (Hall, 1974; Hersen & Barlow, 1976; Sidman, 1960).

The terms *dependent* and *independent* describe the relationship between the two variables. The dependent variable (the communication and language behaviors being measured) "depends" upon the independent variable (Alberto & Troutman, 1982). The independent variable in this case is your implementation of CLIP.

Length of Baseline

There is no definitive statement regarding how many data points are required in order to have an adequate baseline. Alberto and Troutman (1982), Axelrod (1983), and Hall (1974) recommend a minimum of five sessions. However, Alberto and Troutman, Axelrod, and Hall agree that the length of any baseline ultimately depends upon a visual inspection of a graph of the data. In practice, I have found that it is not necessary to spend a great deal of time establishing baselines with individuals who are severely handicapped because more often than not the communication and language behaviors that you want to teach them are simply not present in their repertoires. After three sessions of "0" for percentage correct, begin instructional procedures in the fourth session. However, some moderately to severely handicapped students may respond correctly occasionally but at a very low or inconsistent level. When this occurs, the length of the baseline is determined by both the stability ad the directionality of your data.

STABILITY. A baseline may be considered stable if no data point varies more than 50 percent from the mean or the average of the baseline data (Alberto & Troutman, 1982). For example, if you have collected data for five baseline sessions with correct responding at 15 percent, 25 percent, 20 percent, 15 percent and 10 percent, respectively, the mean is 17 percent. If your criterion is that no response will vary more than 50 percent from the mean, you divide 17 by 2 with the result of 8.5 which you round off to 9. Your criteria for this particular baseline is that no data point can be more than 26 percent (17 + 9) or less than 8 percent (17 − 9). According to the 50 percent rule, this baseline is stable because no data point varies more than 50 percent from the mean. (It is important to note that the criterion for stability is usually much more rigorous for research purposes. Sidman [1960] recommends a 5 percent variability.)

DIRECTIONALITY. Practical considerations and the reality of the erratic responding frequently encountered with moderately to severely handicapped populations may make it seemingly impossible to achieve stable baselines. Consequently, I suggest that anytime there are ten baseline sessions below 50 percent correct responding, the directionality (trend) of the data determines the length of the baseline. When the trend is downward, begin intervention using the instructional procedures described in CLIP. I make this statement with the full realization that there may be many applied behavior analysts who will disagree, but I do so because there are practical considerations involved, not the least of which is that ten baseline data points reflect two weeks' lost teaching time.

For teaching purposes, I also think that it is appropriate to begin intervention procedures after ten sessions that were extremely *erratic,* such as 10 percent one session, 70 percent the next session, then 20 percent, 50 percent and, finally, 20 percent again. Such erratic responding is an indication that the response is in the student's repertoire and, as a language instructor, you want to stabilize correct responding at a high level. When you begin teaching following such an erratic baseline, do so after a particularly poor performance when the trend is downward, rather than when the student appears to be improving without intervention.

The direction of the data is also a factor to consider when determining the length of the baseline. Graphing data provides a picture of whether the behavior of interest is consistently increasing or decreasing (being strengthened or weakened). Since the purpose of communication and language intervention is to *strengthen* these behaviors it is unwise to begin intervention if the baseline data indicate that the communication and language behaviors are improving without intervention. This would be evident by an upward trend or an ascendig basline. One would initiate intervention on an ascending baseline only for behaviors that she wished to weaken (Alberto & Troutman, 1982; Axelrod, 1983; Hall, 1974). Examples of such behaviors would be self-injurious behaviors, self-stimulation, and many forms of echolalia.

Single-Subject Designs

Single-subject designs involve taking repeated measures of the dependent variables during baseline and intervention conditions. These measures are taken on a single subject who, essentially, serves as his or her own experimental control, thus eliminating the problem of finding large numbers of moderately to severely communicatively impaired individuals who have exactly the same communication problem so that they can be assigned randomly to experimental and control groups. Furthermore, it is not necessary for half of your students who would be serving in the control group to go without treatment. Finally, single-subject designs are ideal for individualizing instruction.

Several of these designs are discussed in this chapter, including AB, multiple baseline, reversal, changing criterion, alternating treatments, and changing conditions designs. These designs provide varying degrees of experimental control. The greater the experimental control, the better you have demonstrated your accountability. They also vary as far as the difficulty in implementation and the amount of data required. Advantages and disadvantages of each design will be pointed out.

AB Design

This design reflects two conditions, one baseline and one intervention designated A and B, respectively. This simple design actually forms the basis for all single-subject designs (Alberto & Troutman, 1982). Others refer to it as a simple time-series design (Tawney & Gast, 1984). Data are collected and recorded during the baseline or preintervention phase. Once the baseline is stable and the direction of the data is trending downward (or the data meet other criteria described above under "Length of Baseline"), you can begin to implement your communication and language intervention procedures. Continue recording and graphing data during the intervention phase. These data can then be compared to the baseline data to provide information about the effectiveness of the communication and language intervention.

Figure 4-3 is an example of data collected using an AB design. Notice that the baseline and the intervention phases are separated by a vertical line and that the final data point of the baseline is not connected to the initial data point of the intervention phase (Hall, 1974).

Figure 4-3

GRAPH OF HYPOTHETICAL DATA OF TWO COMMUNICATIVE TASKS
AB DESIGN

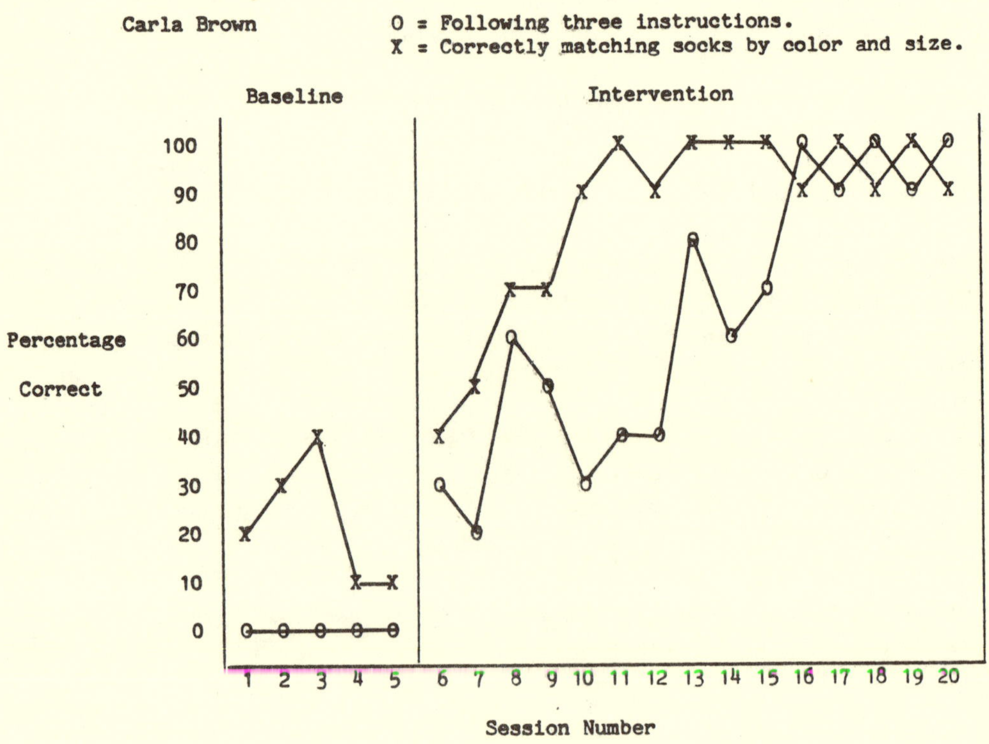

ADVANTAGES. Some of the advantages of this design are obvious. The graph provides an excellent visual presentation of the effects that intervention had on targeted communication and langauge behaviors. The trend of the data provides information regarding the behaviors being measured. It is easy to determine when a student meets criteria on particular tasks so that you know when to start thinning the reinforcement schedule on that task and begin instruction on another. The trend of the data also indicates whether it is necessary to change your intervention procedures, such as using stronger or weaker prompts, varying reinforcers or delivering stronger reinforcers, varying antecedent stimuli, etc., as was discussed in Chapter 3. (However, if you change your intervention procedures, this design would change accordingly to ABCD . . . N.)

DISADVANTAGES. The major disadvantage of an AB design is that you cannot conclude that any positive changes that occurred during the intervention phase was the direct result of that intervention. This design does not control for confounding variables that may have occurred. This simply means that while the data suggest that your instruction was effective, any skeptic could legitimately ask, "How do you know that something else didn't happen at approximately the same point in time as data point number 6?" This is fair criticism. It is possible that any number of confounding variables could have occurred at that point in time or shortly thereafter: The student could have been placed on some medication, the parents may have gotten divorced and the home enviornment improved dramatically, someone else may have started communication instruction at about the same time, or myelinization may have occurred just at that moment! The following procedures are designed to overcome this problem.

Mulitple Baseline Design

You or others may want further evidence regarding the effectiveness of your teaching procedures. You can provide this clearly by using any one of a number of single-subject research designs. A multiple baseline design is particularly popular with educators and speech-language pathologists. A multiple baseline permits you to determine the effects of your instruction (the independent variable) on more than one dependent variable at the same time. Thus, a multiple baseline procedure can be applied to two or more behaviors (tasks), the same behavior in two or more situations or settings, or to the same behavior with two or more students (Alberto & Troutman, 1982; Axelrod, 1983; Baer, Wolf, & Risley, 1968; Hall, 1974; Hersen & Barlow, 1976; Tawney & Gast, 1984).

A multiple baseline procedure that involves collecting data on several different tasks (target behaviors) that you are going to teach a student is highly recommended. Since CLIP normally involves working on at least three to five different tasks during each session, this would simply extend the baseline phases for two to four of them. In other words, you would begin collecting and recording baseline data on, say, three tasks. Then you would begin your intervention or teaching procedures on one task, that is, you would provide reinforcers, prompts, etc., as described in Chapter 3, in order for the student to master the task. However, you would keep collecting baseline data on the other two tasks without starting any teaching procedures on them until the first task reaches the predetermined criteria. Then you would start the same teaching procedures on the second task while continuing to keep baseline data on the third task. When the second task also reaches criteria, you would implement the teaching procedures on the third task.

I also recommend using a multiple baseline procedure on the same behavior across two or more situations or settings. Here again, CLIP is designed so that students are instructed in at least three different settings, preferably school, home, and community. To collect data across settings, you simply begin collecting data in two or more settings. When the baseline data are stable or meet other criteria described under "Length of Baseline," begin intervention in one of the settings and continue collecting data under baseline conditions in the other setting(s). As the student reaches criterion in the intervention setting, begin intervention in the next setting, and so on until intervention is occurring in all settings or the student has generalized correct responding at criterion level in settings where no training had occurred and, therefore, training in those settings is unnecessary.

It is possible to use a multiple baseline treatment across two or more individuals also. However, I do not recommend this procedure as highly as across behaviors or settings because you have lost one of the most positive advantages of single-subject research designs since the subject no longer serves as his or her own experimental control. Nevertheless, there may be circumstances when you determine that you can afford that loss. If so, the procedure is similar to those described above. You would select a particular communication or language task that you wanted to teach to two or more students. After getting a stable baseline measure on all of them, you would then introduce instruction sequentially on each of the remaining students. As the first student reaches criteria, you begin instructing the second while the third remains in baseline conditions, and so forth until all of the students are receiving instruction.

ADVANTAGES. The advantages of this procedure are many. As you can see, this sequential treatment across tasks, settings, or individuals provides excellent evidence that your teaching procedures are responsible for the student's learning. Everything else in his environment was the same. That is, he was growing and developing, his diet or medication varied or stayed the same, his parents were getting along well or fighting, he was in a good mood or a bad mood when he got to school, etc. However, one thing and only one thing was deliberately manipulated by you, and that was whether you would provide him with reinforcing consequences, prompts, etc., on a particular communication or langauge task while not on other tasks or on a particular communication or language task in certain settings and not in other settings, or you would reinforce him as a particular student and not reinforce other students. Thus, you can demonstrate the functional relationship between your instruction and your student's learning. Furthermore, you can do so without stopping instruction, as is necessary in the following reversal design; therefore, parents, administrators, and others are very receptive to a multiple baseline procedure.

DISADVANTAGES. However, there are limitations to a multiple baseline procedure. The most serious limitation I have experienced is that some behaviors are interdependent. That is, intervention on one effects a change on others, making it impossible to demonstrate conclusively what caused the behavioral change. It is also necessary for those communication and language behaviors in the baseline conditions to go without instruction until there is evidence of mastery in the previous intervention condition, or for a student to go without instruction in certain settings until a particular communicative behavior has been mastered in prior settings. Or, when used across students, those students who are in the baseline conditions do not receive instruction for, occasionally, quite extended periods of time. Another difficulty I have encountered with a multiple baseline procedure is the amount of data collection required. Remember, once you start collecting the data across two or more behaviors, settings, or students, you must continue to collect it until you have replicated your instructional procedures across all of them. Furthermore, multiple baselines across students require similar individuals with similar learning histories; and multiple baselines across behaviors require behaviors that are independent of each other, yet responsive to the same independent variable(s).

Nevertheless, I feel that the advantages of this design are so powerful that they outweigh the disadvantages, and the multiple settings, as well as the recommended multiple communication and language tasks simultaneously trained in CLIP, are ideal for using a multiple baseline procedure. Normally, when a multiple baseline procedure is applied to one behavior across two or more settings, instruction occurs and data are collected in specific settings daily or at set intervals (e.g., math and reading sessions) (Ayllon, Layman, & Kandel, 1975). However, CLIP is designed for training in three major settings: home, school and community. Plan to collect data in specific settings in the home and school settings. However, it is highly unlikely that identical community settings will be readily available on a daily basis. Therefore, a setting schedule similar to the following is recommended:

1. Billy's father will instruct Billy and take data at home at the kitchen table each evening after dinner.
2. Ms. Scheckenberg will instruct Billy and take data between 10:00 and 10:30 A.M. in the classroom setting each weekday.

3. Mr. Abnernathy will instruct Billy and collect data between 2:00 and 2:30 P.M. each weekday at the park, the laundromat, the grocery store, the bowling alley, the drug store, or wherever the daily community training occurs.

It is only necessary to collect data for 10 or 20 trials per session in each of these three settings. Therefore, there is minimal, if any, interruption in the ongoing activities. For example, the particular task for the hypothetical data in Figure 4-4 is the ability to follow three instructions. It would be very easy for Mr. Abernathy and Billy's father to record Billy's response to any of several three-part instructions natural to the home and community environments.

If a student begins to use communication and language skills in some of the nontrained settings or, better still, on communicative tasks that have not received training, you have evidence that he is generalizing appropriately, which is one of the major objectives of this program. However, if this generalization occurs before intervention in at least two settings, there is no evidence that these instructional procedures effected the positive change in his communication and language behaviors. The following graph depicts hypothetical data on a multiple baseline design across three settings:

Figure 4-4

GRAPH OF HYPOTHETICAL DATA ON FOLLOWING INSTRUCTIONS
MULTIPLE BASELINE DESIGN ACROSS THREE SETTINGS

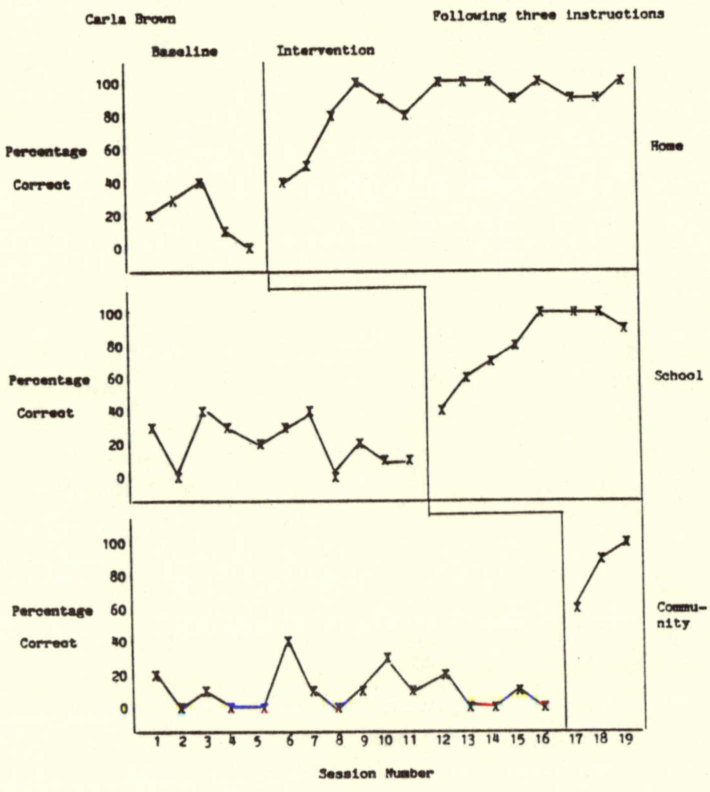

Reversal Design

A reversal design is another good way to determine whether your instruction was effective or not. However, I do not recommend it as highly as the multiple baseline because I have found that it is frequently very difficult for teachers to implement because it involves returning to baseline conditions where no teaching occurs. In other words, you take the baseline on the communication task of interest, then you implement the teaching procedures just as you would if you were doing a multiple baseline. When the student reaches criteria on the task, you return to baseline conditions by withdrawing all instructional procedures, such as reinforcing correct responses and correcting incorrect responses. Quite logically, a reversal design that implements these three phases is often referred to as an ABA design. If the student has been reinforced on a continuous (CRF) or very dense fixed-ratio (e.g., FR 2) reinforcement schedule, her correct responding normally will return to baseline level quickly, or at least drop off considerably. You can then reinstitute intervention procedures in order to reestablish a high level of appropriate communication and language behaviors. When this is done, the four phases are referred to as an ABAB design (Alberto & Troutman, 1982; Axelrod, 1983; Hall, 1974; Tawney & Gast, 1984).

ADVANTAGES. The obvious advantage of a reversal procedure is its simplicity. The systematic replication of the baseline and intervention phases provides a precise analysis of the effects of independent variable (the communication and language intervention of the language instructor) had on the dependent variable (the communication and language behaviors of the student) (Sidman, 1960). Another advantage of a reversal as opposed to a multiple baseline procedure is that, normally, it doesn't take as long to get evidence about the effectiveness of your teaching procedures, nor does it involve such extensive data collection. Furthermore, as soon as the behavior drops off or returns to baseline during a reversal procedure, you should reinstitute your teaching procedures immediately; otherwise, using this design could be considered unethical or unprofessional (Alberto & Troutman, 1982).

DISADVANTAGES. One of the major disadvantages is that withdrawing instruction may be difficult for teachers to do. Once we have taught a student something, we don't want to see him lose it. Furthermore, some behaviors appear to be irreversible, and communication and language behaviors are very likely to fall into that category. Once a person learns how to communicate effectively, it is highly unlikely that simply removing positive consequences will cause him to *unlearn* such behaviors. There are also ethical considerations related to introducing a reversal procedure after eliminating dangerous or extremely inappropriate behaviors. While such behaviors are not the direct focus of this program, it is not uncommon for inappropriate behaviors to weaken or even disappear when appropriate behaviors (such as communicating effectively) are strengthened (Allyon, Layman & Kandel, 1975). Just as with a multiple baseline technique, this kind of systematic replication is the ultimate test of whether your teaching procedures are, in fact, responsible for the student's learning. Figure 4-5 is an example of a graph which shows a reversal procedure.

Figure 4-5

GRAPH OF HYPOTHETICAL DATA OF ABILITY TO GENERATE THREE-WORD SENTENCES
ABAB REVERSAL DESIGN

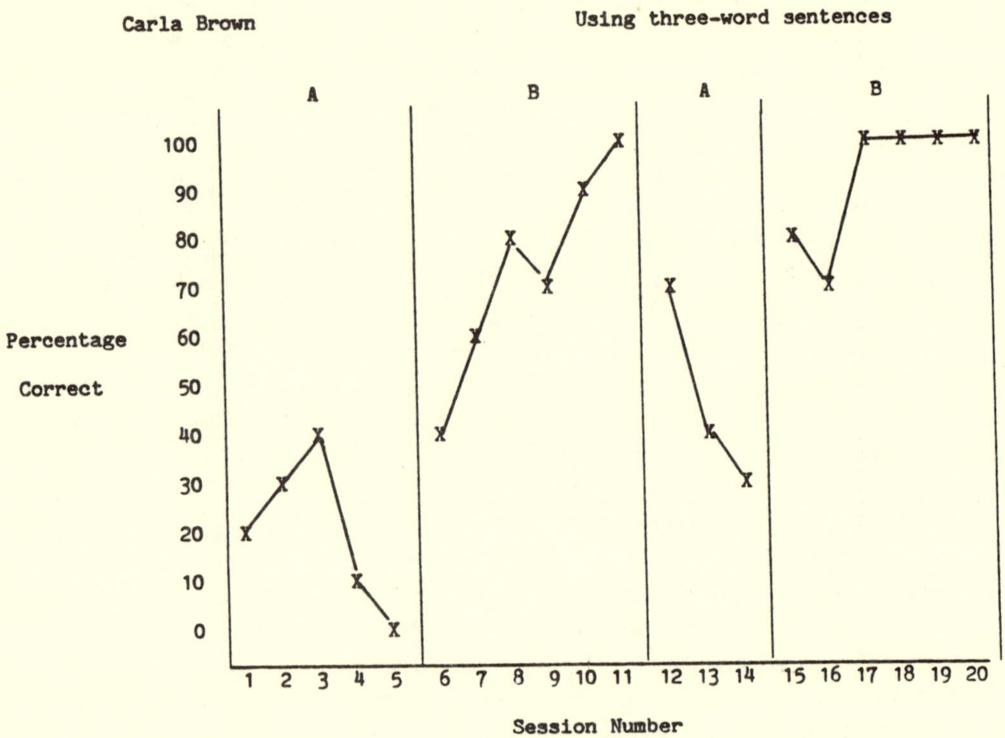

Changing Criterion Design

The changing criterion design is a variation of the multiple baseline design (Hall & Fox, 1977). It may be one of the most useful with the severely communicatively handicapped population because it is one which is particularly appropriate when reaching the terminal behavior will take a considerable length of time (Alberto & Troutman, 1982) and it is particularly suited to demonstrating the effectiveness of shaping procedures (Hall, 1974; Hall & Fox, 1977; Hartmann & Hall, 1976). As you recall from chapter 3, shaping behavior requires gradually changing the performance level of the behavior you will reinforce.

The changing criterion design, while a variation of the multiple baseline design, requires that each treatment phase is associated with a step-wise change in the criterion for the behavior you are measuring (Alberto & Troutman, 1982; Hall, 1974; Hall & Fox, 1977; Hartmann & Hall, 1976; Tawney & Gast, 1984). Essentially, each phase of this design provides a baseline for the following phase. As the rate of the communicative behavior you are measuring changes with each step-wise change in the criterion, instructional procedures are replicated and the cause-effect relationship between the instructional procedures and the communicatively handicapped individual's improved responding is demonstrated.

This design is implemented in essentially the same manner as a reversal or multiple baseline design in that you begin by taking baseline data. After the baseline is established, you must determine the criterion or the required level of the targeted behavior in the next phase. This is usually based on the mean level of responding in the baseline phase, but, in any event, it should be well within the student's capabilities (Hall & Fox, 1977). This can be done by setting the criterion at or near the mean (Hall & Fox, 1977) or 50 percent above the mean of the baseline data (Alberto & Troutman, 1982). For example, if you are instructing the student in syntax and morphology, one of the objectives is to gradually increase the length of sentences to five to seven words. Thus, if your recorded spontaneous language samples reveal that the student's average sentence length is two words, the criterion for the first intervention phase would be three words. During this phase, you only reinforce the student for using sentences of at least three words. Continuing with this logic, the criterion for the next phase would be four-and-one-half words, which, of course, is normally impossible. Therefore, I would recommend a criterion of four words for phase 3. Finally, the criterion for phase 4 would be six words.

ADVANTAGES. A functional relationship between instruction and learning is indicated if the data reflect that the student's behavior corresponds to the predetermined criterion in each phase. An obvious advantage of the changing criterion design is that you can demonstrate the functional relationship between your teaching and the student's learning without withdrawing your instructional procedures. Therefore, changes in student behavior are always in a positive direction.

DISADVANTAGES. A possible disadvantage is that the design requires very gradual behavior changes. Consequently, you may be holding some students back. For instance, considering the example given above, it is possible that when the criterion was set at four words in phase 3, the student could have been producing five- or six-word sentences. Another disadvantage is that demonstrating a functional relationship between the student's learning and your instructional procedures depends upon how accurately you predict each successive criterion level. Furthermore, use of the changing criterion design should be restricted to behaviors that are already present in a student's communicative repertoire which you wish to strengthen or stabilize. It is not an appropriate design for the initial acquisition of communicative behaviors.

Nevertheless, this is a nice variation of the multiple baseline design, retaining most of the advantages of that design with the added advantage of requiring considerably less data collection. It is particularly advantageous when instructing moderately to severely handicapped populations because it is the only design which systematically corresponds to shaping procedures in the sense of gradually strengthening (or, in some cases, weakening) behaviors that are already present in a student's behavioral repertoire. Figure 4-6 provides an example of a changing criterion design.

Figure 4-6

GRAPH OF HYPOTHETICAL DATA OF TIME ON TASK
CHANGING CRITERION DESIGN

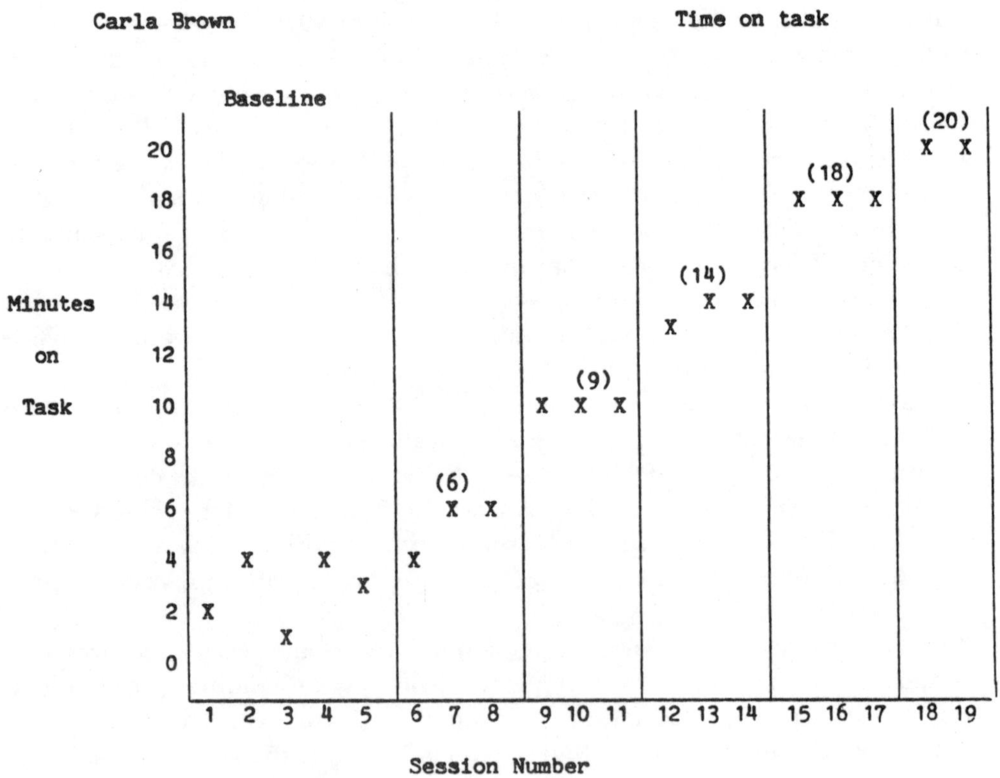

Numbers in parentheses indicate criterion set at each successive phase.

Alternating Treatments Design

This particular single-subject design goes by many names: multielement design (Axelrod, 1983), multielement baseline design (Sidman, 1960), multiple schedule design (Hersen & Barlow, 1976), and alternating treatments design (Alberto & Troutman, 1982; Barlow & Hayes, 1979; Barrera & Sulzer-Azaroff, 1983; Tawney & Gast, 1984). I have chosen to use the latter term because it seems to be the most descriptive. According to Alberto and Troutman, the design can be used in two ways:

1. Comparing the effects of two or more instructional procedures after taking baseline data.
2. Comparing the effects of two or more instructional procedures with a control (no instruction) condition. This control condition is the equivalent of a baseline condition that is maintained throughout the investigation.

In the first procedure, begin by taking baseline data just as in any of the previously described designs. Then identify two or more instructional procedures and set up an implementation schedule. Alberto and Troutman (1982) recommend exposing the student to each instructional procedure an equal number of times, while systematically rotating the order of the procedures. For example, if you have three instructional procedures, the following orders of presentations are possible: XYZ, YZX, ZXY, XZY, YXZ, and ZYX. Use each order of procedures at least once and avoid schedules that would allow one procedure to be used twice in succession without an intervening procedure, such as following the first XYZ schedule by the ZXY schedule, thus repeating Z.

In the second procedure, you may choose to initiate two or more instructional procedures and take repeated measures on them while continuing to record data in a baseline condition (Alberto & Troutman, 1982). You are comparing two or more treatments with a no treatment or control condition. Alberto, Jobes, Sizemore, and Doran (1980) used this procedure to compare individual and group instruction across response tasks.

A third variation of this procedure consists of two or more instructors alternating instructional procedures (Doke & Risley, 1972; O'Brien, Azrin, & Henson, 1969; Redd & Birnbrauer, 1969). This is a nice procedure to control for the effects of unique teacher traits, thus gaining a more distinct picture of the effects of the instructional procedures.

ADVANTAGES. One of the advantages of this design is that several instructional procedures can be compared quickly. It does not require withdrawing instructional procedures which usually results in a reversal of educational gains. It is also particularly useful when the behaviors under consideration are interdependent which overcomes one of the serious difficulties with the multiple baseline design. Furthermore, if you compare the effects of the instructional procedures with a control condition, you have the advantage of being able to proceed with your instruction immediately without waiting until you have collected traditional baseline data.

DISADVANTAGES. One of the disadvantages of this design, particularly for the student population we are concerned with, is that it is necessary to demonstrate differences in treatment conditions almost immediately. This requires students who are able to understand which treatment is in effect in order to respond differentially immediately. The major disadvantage is the failure of this design to establish a functional relationship between instructional procedures and learning. Although the instructional procedures are alternated and appear, on the surface, to be very much like an ABAB reversal design, the effect one instructional procedure may have on the same behaviors in another instructional condition cannot be determined. However, this disadvantage is much more applicable for researchers than for educators. See Figure 4-7 for a graph of hypothetical data depicting two language instructors alternating instructional procedures to determine the effects on their young communicatively impaired students' ability to ask questions.

Figure 4-7

GRAPH OF HYPOTHETICAL DATA OF NUMBER OF QUESTIONS ASKED
PHASES ALTERNATED BETWEEN INSTRUCTORS AND INSTRUCTIONAL PROCEDURES
ALTERNATING TREATMENTS DESIGN

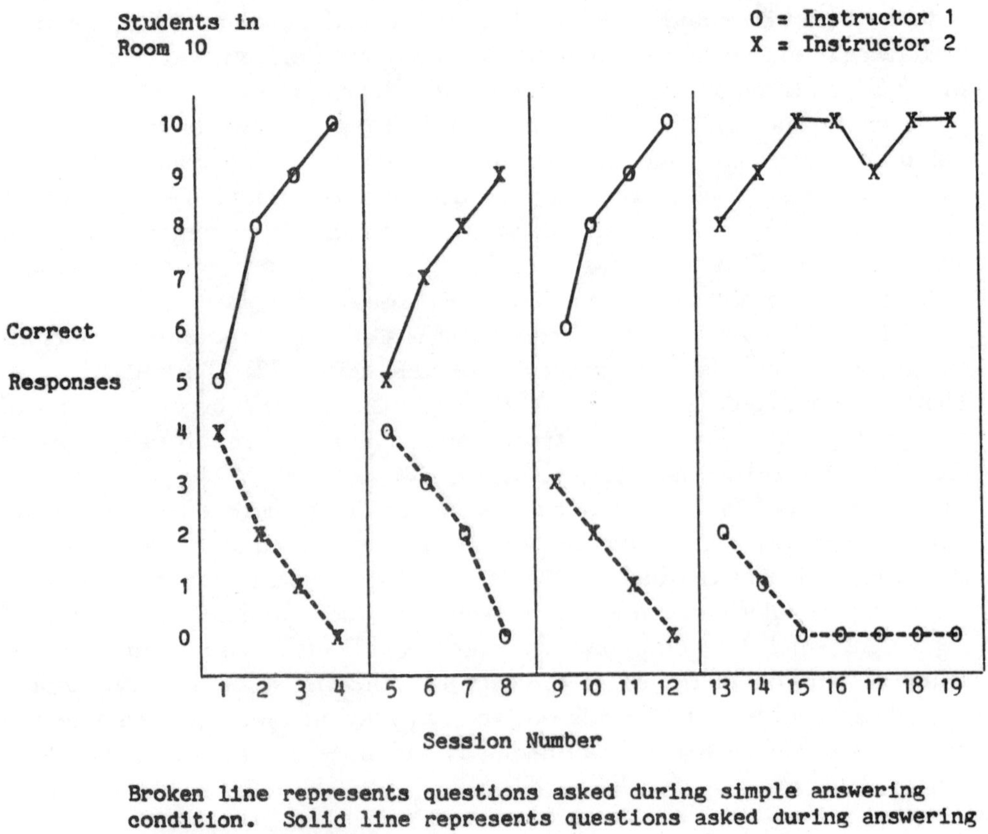

Broken line represents questions asked during simple answering condition. Solid line represents questions asked during answering and praising condition.

Changing Conditions Design

This design is simply an extension of the AB design. In the changing conditions design two or more instructional procedures are introduced after establishing a stable baseline or otherwise meeting the conditions described under "Length of Baseline." This design reflects the reality of educational settings, in that language instructors and others try different instructional procedures until they find one that works (Alberto & Troutman, 1982).

If the data in the first instructional phase do not indicate student improvement, a second procedure is introduced, and so on until your data provide evidence that your instructional procedure is effective. Thus, the design could be ABCD . . . N, implementing as many different instructional approaches as are required to find one that is successful. Each letter represents a different procedure.

Figure 4-8

GRAPH OF HYPOTHETICAL DATA ON NUMBER OF QUESTIONS STUDENTS ASKED
CHANGING CONDITIONS DESIGN

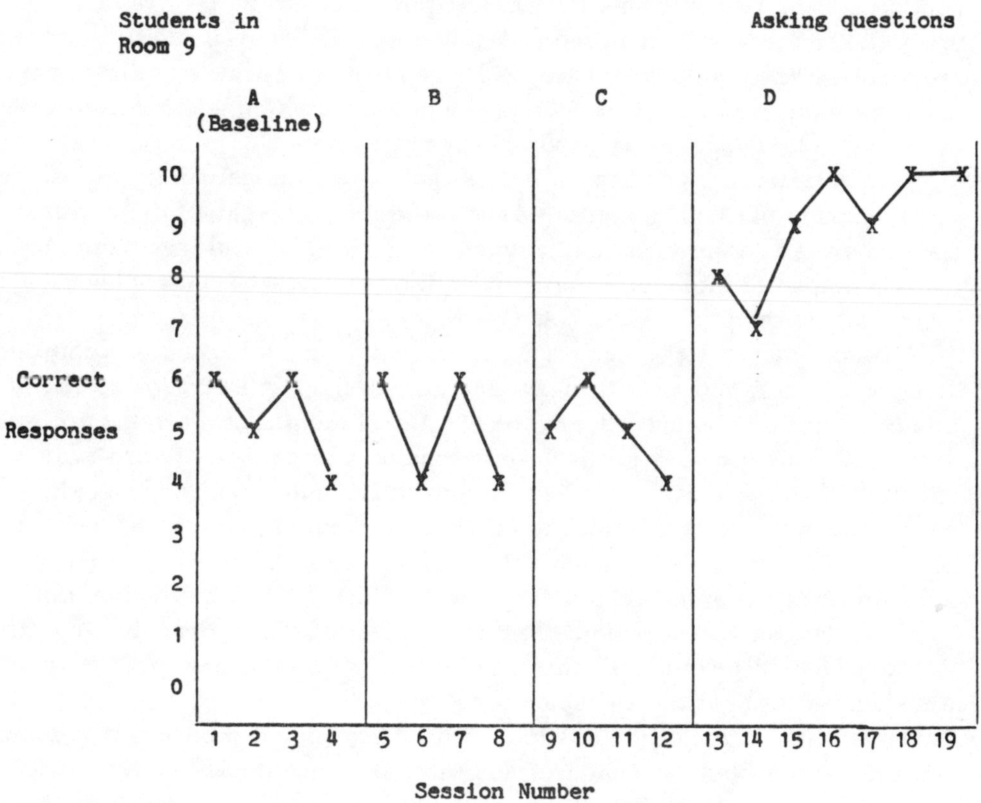

ADVANTAGES. One of the advantages of this design is that it is ideal for the instructor who finds it necessary to try several different approaches before finding one that is successful. Also, keeping and graphing data for each instructional procedure make it possible to determine whether the procedure is effective.

DISADVANTAGES. Although you do have a systematic record of student performance, this design does not provide evidence of a functional relationship between an instructional procedure and learning that occurs. This disadvantage could be overcome quite easily by implementing a return-to-baseline condition. Figure 4-8 is a graphic display of hypothetical data on students asking questions using a changing conditions design.

Putting Standardized Tests to Good Use

While I strongly urge instructors to use a single-subject design that is appropriate to their particular situation, the standardized communication and language tests that are usually required by local, state, and/or federal lesgislation in order to identify students who are communicatively impaired can be put to good use, also. This section sets forth an approach to using the pre- and post-test data that are usually required and, therefore, readily available. It is written especially for those who have tried, as I have, to demonstrate significant gains made by moderately to severely handicapped students on standardized communication, language, or psycholinguistic tests.

First, it is necessary to determine communication and language acquisition up to the point in time the pretest was administered. This can be done with any test that gives a communication, language, or psycholinguistic age score. Then convert that score into months and divide it by the student's chronological age on the date of the pretest, also converted into months.

Second, when the post-tests are administered, use the same procedure to convert the communication, language or psycholinguistic age score into months. Then divide that score by the number of months between the pre- and post-tests. This provides for an intraindividual comparison of each student's communication and language acquisition before and after receiving the instructional procedures described in CLIP. It is essential that students begin receiving instruction immediately after the pretest. Otherwise, there is a misrepresentation of the time period during which they received communication and language instruction. The intraindividual scores can be analyzed statistically to determine whether changes in communication and language were significant by using a simple t test.

ADVANTAGES. One of the advantages of using this procedure is that something is learned from the standardized tests that wasn't already evident, assuming that most people are aware that an individual who has moderate to severe communication or language impairments does, indeed, have the problem, and tests simply confirm this commonsense judgment. Another advantage is that you can provide administrators and others with data which more fairly reflect the effectiveness of your instructional procedures.

DISADVANTAGES. A disadvantage is the necessity of implementing the instructional procedures immediately after the pretests are administered. This may be difficult in situations where one or a few communication and language instructors are responsible for testing and delivering services to many students. On the other hand, realizing that every day between the pretest and the day service delivery begins negatively affects the amount of improvement demonstrated, may provide an impetus to complete the testing very quickly or arrange for instructional procedures with students who have been tested to go on simultaneously with testing remaining students. Another disadvantage is that there is valid skepticism about the efficacy of using these procedures becaue there is no control for possible confounding variables that may have occurred concurrently during the instructional period. However, once again, this may be a serious disadvantage for reseachers but have little consequence for parents, teachers, and others.

SUMMARY

This chapter has provided information regarding how to collect and record data. *Data* is a term that most parents, teachers, and speech pathologists usually leave to the experts. However, as Hall (1971) pointed out, parents and teachers can implement many of these research designs quite simply, and they can do so in natural home and educational environments.

I do not feel that it is necessary to use one of the single-subject designs on every task you teach a student. But it is extremely reinforcing for *you* if you do so periodically. It will provide you with some certainty about the effectiveness of your instructional procedures. The data revealed by these designs also provide extremely useful information to share with administrators and others about your accountability.

Systematic replication of instructional procedures and consequent learning is the ultimate test of cause-effect relationships between these independent and dependent variables (Baer, Wolf, & Risley, 1968; Sidman, 1960). Therefore, it is the ultimate test of whether your instructional procedures are, in fact, responsible for your students' learning.

CHAPTER 5

GENERALIZATION

JANE Y. MURDOCK

PERHAPS the ultimate test for how well you have succeeded in teaching a severely communicatively impaired individual is related to how well he generalizes what he has learned, as well as how long those behaviors persist. This includes both stimulus generalization and response generalization. In order to determine this, you must investigate stimulus generalization to determine whether he uses what he has learned (1) in other *physical settings,* (2) with other *people*, and (3) in response to different *discriminative stimuli,* that is, the visual, auditory and tactile signals you present to the student in order to evoke the response. You must also investigate response generalization by determining (4) whether he responds appropriately on *other language tasks* that are similar to those which he has been taught specifically (Murdock & Hartmann, 1975).

PLANNING FOR GENERALIZATION

The following discussion of generalization is based on a review of generalization literature written by Trevor F. Stokes and Donald M. Baer. The techniques are restricted to those used in applied behavior analysis research. Stokes and Baer (1977, p. 350) categorized techniques designed to assess or program generalization according to nine general headings:

1. Train and hope
2. Sequential modification
3. Introduce to natural maintaining contingencies
4. Train sufficient exemplars
5. Train loosely
6. Use indiscriminable contingencies
7. Program common stimuli

8. Mediate generalization
9. Train "to generalize"

Train and Hope

This is the most common technique used to assess generalization. After the student has mastered targeted communicative behaviors, there is some follow-up testing or observations implemented to determine whether generalization of those behaviors occurred across settings, experimenters, responses, and time.

The train-and-hope technique is just that: You train the behaviors and hope that they will generalize. According to Stokes and Baer (1977), this technique makes up about half of the applied literature on generalization. While about 90 percent of the train-and-hope studies reported successful generalization, according to Stokes and Baer much of this could be the result of limited investigations and/or failure on the part of researchers to include the topic of generalization in their reports when it failed to occur.

Sequential Modification

Sequential modification involves more than simply assessing whether generalization occurred or not. If the assessment reveals that generalization is not occurring or is not occurring consistently, procedures are initiated to attempt to promote generalization. These usually involve introducing the original instructional procedures in every relevant generalization situation. A student is presented with appropriate discriminative stimuli and provided feedback in the form of correction or reinforcement, depending upon her responses.

Introduce Natural Maintaining Contingencies

This is the ideal generalization technique, and it is involved from the moment CLIP is implemented because the emphasis is on teaching in natural environments throughout the students' waking hours. Natural maintaining contingencies are further exemplified when the behaviors being taught are immediately functional for the student and, thus, are naturally reinforced. It is important to be sensitive to natural maintaining contingencies since these frequently are responsible for poor communication and language skills, as well as other inappropriate behaviors (e.g., the student who is rarely required to speak because parents, teachers, and others assume that he cannot do so and they anticipate his every wish). When situations such as this exist, arrangements have to be made to rearrange the environment so that the student is required to use the communicative behaviors that he has.

Training Sufficient Exemplars

This technique is described in Chapter 3 under "How to Establish Specific Language Structures." It may be necessary for a moderately to severely communicatively impaired student to master many, many exemplars of the plural form, for example, before he makes the necessary inductions for appropriate generalization to nontrained plurals. This applies to both regular and irregular forms. The same is true of all morphological forms, phonology, and syntax.

According to Stokes and Baer (1977), this is the most extensively reported generalization technique in the applied behavior analysis literature, and it is possibly one of the most valuable areas for programming. The procedures involve training *sufficient* exemplars in order to accomplish generalization to untrained situations and responses as opposed to training in every relevant situation. Thus, it appears that probing for new responses, in different settings, and with other people not involved in the training would have to continue until appropriate generalization occurred. However, in practice, other experimenters frequently become involved in the training in order to facilitate the generalization, and probing and training also occur in other physical settings (Allen, 1973; Garcia, 1974; Handleman, 1979; Hurlbut, Iwata, & Green, 1982; McGee, Krantz, Mason, & McClannahan, 1983; Murdock, Garcia, & Hardman, 1977; Stokes, Baer, & Jackson, 1974).

Train Loosely

This is the most simple and informal technique, in that there is a concerted effort not to control the stimuli presented and the responses allowed. Stokes and Baer suggest that this approach might be conceptualized as negating the discrimination technique. While the one research effort they reported suggests that training loosely results in greater generalization than tightly restricted models, this is difficult to investigate extensively because of the rigorous demands placed upon replicable research. If the milieu-type instruction recommended in CLIP is implemented, however, extensive concurrent training should occur automatically.

Use Nondiscriminable Contingencies

Thinning reinforcement schedules to unpredictable, intermittent schedules has been emphasized throughout CLIP because behaviors maintained on such schedules are highly resistant to extinction. In effect, this results in generalization over time. If students are reinforced in a variety of settings by a variety of people, on an unpredictable reinforcement schedule, it appears that they would also generalize across settings and people. There is some evidence that delayed reinforcement also has a positive effect on generalization. Stokes and Baer speculate that this may be a result of failure to discriminate the contingencies. According to Stokes and Baer (1977, p. 358):

> In general, it may be suspected that delayed reinforcement often will have the advantage of making the times and places in which the contingency actually operates indiscriminable to the subject. However, this advantage is an advantage, by hypothesis, primarily for the goal of generalization. Otherwise, delayed reinforcement would often be considered an inefficient technique, most especially so for the initial development of a new skill. Indeed, it may be exactly in the realm of disadvantaged persons such as retarded children that the usual inefficiency of delayed reinforcement may seem the most severe handicap to its use. However, its potential for fostering generalization suggests strongly that further research be invested in this procedure (and any others that make reinforcement contingencies properly indiscriminable), to develop methods of applying it perhaps only after the initial development of a new skill, in the interests of promoting generalization.

Considering the communication and language acquisition problems experienced by moderately to severely communicatively impaired students, it would not appear wise to attempt to promote generalization by presenting nondiscernible contingencies since there is good evidence that doing so delays initial acquisition. Furthermore, in all probability, there is enough nondiscernible contingency management going on in the natural environments of many of those we are concerned with that any positive effects it may have on generalization will be accomplished, if not precisely measurable for publishable research.

Program Common Stimuli

There is some evidence that stimuli common to the training setting and the generalization settings effect generalization positively. These common stimuli can be people, furniture, teaching materials, etc. There is considerable evidence that if peers are present in both the training and generalization settings, generalization is enhanced. A little thought about student behavior during the presence or absence of certain individuals (e.g., the principal or a substitute teacher) provides further evidence of the effect people may have on generalization. The same holds true for any stimuli that are common to both the training and the generalization environments. Stokes and Baer conclude (1977, pp. 36-37): "A common stimulus approach to generalization would encourage the incorporation into training settings of (naturally occurring) physical stimuli that are frequently prominent or functional in nontraining environments. If these stimuli are well chosen and can be made functional and salient in the training procedures, then generalization may thereby be programmed."

If parents, teachers, paraprofessionals, siblings, and others assume an instructional role (as is recommended in CLIP), there will be abundant opportunities for common, functional stimuli to be present in a variety of settings without careful programming.

Mediate Generalization

Mediated generalization is often used to explain the ability of individuals to generalize rather abstract concepts to new learning. It may be the essence of some of the definitions of creativity, such as coming up with new ideas by putting old ideas into new combinations. According to Stokes and Baer (1977), the most common mediator is probably language. The generalization, therefore, is not of the communication or language per se but rather using language to mediate nonverbal behaviors in a variety of situations. Stokes and Baer state (1977, p. 363):

> It may be reasonable to suggest that in the development of language-training programs, systematic attention be given to the training of language skills sufficiently well elaborated to function as mediators of nonverbal behavior. Language is a response, of course; it is also, equally obviously, a stimulus to the speaker as well as to the listener. Thus it meets perfectly the logic of a salient common stimulus, to be carried from any training setting to any generalization setting that the child may ever enter. It also perfectly exemplifies the active generalization approach recommended earlier.

One of the objectives of CLIP is to teach students to use communication and language to control their own behavior and the behavior of others.

Train to Generalize

In their discussion of generalization techniques, Stokes and Baer (1977) are considering generalization itself as a response that, conceivably, could be contingently reinforced. This might be accomplished without specifically instructing or otherwise cueing a student simply by reinforcing her whenever she demonstrates that she is generalizing her communicative behaviors in increasingly sophisticated forms.

There are many examples of this, ranging from using signs at the grocery store that are normally used only in the therapy setting, to generalizing from American Sign Language with its particular syntactic structure to perfectly spoken English syntax. Furthermore, if we are training generalization, it is appropriate to use instructions to facilitate it. If a student has mastered communicative behaviors but is not generalizing optimally, tell him what you want him to do and reinforce him for doing so, at least in the beginning, and gradually thin the reinforcement schedule until naturally occurring reinforcers maintain the communicative behaviors.

GENERALIZATION PROCEDURES WHEN TRAINING IS IN ISOLATED ENVIRONMENTS

Common sense suggests that if communication and language instruction occur in the natural school, home, community, and recreational environments, many of the generalization difficulties we have found with moderately to severely communicatively impaired populations could be avoided. Consequently, our strongest recommendation is to teach communicatively impaired individuals in the setting where that particular communication is needed. Furthermore, the persons doing the teaching ideally will be those individuals who normally interact in that environment, such as parents and siblings in the home; speech and language pathologists, teachers, paraprofessionals, or peers at school; and some combination of all of the above in the community, recreational, and prevocational and vocational environments.

Unfortunately, restrictive regulations, liability insurance policies, fear, outmoded pedagogy, as well as expedience and accountability requirements, frequently make this ideal teaching extremely difficult if not impossible. It often appears to be the rule rather than the exception for speech and language pathologists to provide communication and language instruction to severely impaired students on a one-to-one basis in a more or less isolated setting. While we wish that this were not so, we also wish to provide procedures that will optimize the possibility that both stimulus and reponse generalization will occur anyway.

For example, assume a teaching/learning environment that is probably one of the least conducive to optimal generalization. The communication and language instructor is working with a student in an isolated setting such as her office. The instructor points to a picture of two beds and asks, "What are these?" The student responds correctly by saying, "Beds."

In order to have the four kinds of generalization described above, the student would also have to be able to respond correctly to (1) the same picture and question when asked in a different physical setting such as the classroom or home, (2) the same picture and question when asked by someone other than the language instructor, (3) several different, actual beds, rather than a picture when he is asked the identical question or a variation of the question, and (4) demonstrate his mastery of this plural form to other plurals in which the /z/ phoneme is the plural marker (e.g., chairs, hands, eyes). This last generalization — generalization to other similar language tasks — involves the ability to generalize to different vocabularly words when morphology (word form) and syntax (word order) are involved. Consequently, the student should be able to use plural forms, past tenses, etc., in grammatically correct form as a result of generalizing from similar previously trained words, phrases, and sentences without having received any specific training on them.

Generalization Probing

Probing or testing for generalization should be done for each task as soon as the student gives five to ten consecutive correct responses, or succeeds at 80 percent or better, for two consecutive sessions with the communication and language instructor without prompting after reinforcement has been thinned to at least a VR 5 schedule. In order to determine whether the student's language behaviors are generalizing, the instructor should set up probes to test for each kind of generalization. When probing, approximately four trials are presented for each task without reinforcement. Use the generalization training and probing card in Figure 5-1 for this purpose.

Figure 5-1

GENERALIZATION TRAINING AND PROBING CARD*

Student ____________________ Criteria for correct response:

Date ____________________

Setting / Trainer-Prober	Discriminative Stimuli (Trainer-Prober) Verbal and visual stimuli, prompt, and correction procedures.	Response (Student) Correct (+) Incorrect (-) Prompted correct (p+) Prompted incorrect (p-) No response (0)				Reinforcer and Reinforcement Schedule

1. When probing: Communication-language instructor will fill in verbal and visual stimuli. Trainer-prober will present stimuli four times and record student's responses. Do not reinforce, model, or otherwise prompt.
2. When training: Communication-language instructor will fill in verbal and visual stimuli, prompt, and correction procedures to be used, as well as the reinforcer and the reinforcement schedule. Trainer-prober will present stimuli four times, recording the student's responses and reinforcing or prompting appropriately.
3. The trainer-prober will return these cards to the communication-language instructor daily so that data can be analyzed and appropriate cards prepared for the student's next training-probing session.

*Adapted from Murdock and Hartmann (1975).

1. For generalization to other *physical settings,* the communication and language instructor simply seeks out the student in any setting other than the one in which the language instruction occurred and presents her with the same visual and verbal stimuli. Where the probing occurs makes little difference, as long as it is someplace other than in the initial instructional setting. Ideally, it will be accomplished in the home, school, and community environments. But, minimally, it will be in the classroom, the lunchroom, the hallway, or on the playground.
2. For generalization to other *people,* the communication and language instructor gives a generalization training and probing card to someone else and instructs him or her to present the same visual and verbal stimuli to the student and accurately report her responses. Precise instructions will be on the card. Any person other than the one who did the original language instruction can do this probing. Ideally, it will be done by parents, teachers, paraprofessionals, and others who interact with the student on a regular basis.
3. For generalization to different *discriminative stimuli*, vary the antecedent visual and/or the verbal stimuli on the generalization training and probing cards, still requiring the same response. You might say, "Who is that?" while pointing to her mother who is across the room, rather than "Who is this?" while pointing to a picture of the student's mother you are using for training. Or, when you know the student's mother brought her to school, you might ask, "Who brought you to school today?"
4. Generalization to *similar tasks* can be more difficult to probe for. For example, students should learn to generalize phonemes they have mastered to words they are working on. Until the student has a relatively large vocabulary to work with, new words which utilize the same phonemes or sounds will probably have to be trained independently. However, the student should reach criteria in considerably fewer and fewer trials as new vocabulary is mastered.

When teaching morphological and syntactic structures in Chapter 3, probes for similar task generalization of syntax or word order are required as soon as the student has a two-word combination in her verbal repertoire such as, "More ________." For example, if the student has this chain, you can test her ability to generalize the use of this phrase by presenting her with a visual stimulus for any noun in her vocabulary while phrasing a question which indicates that she is to respond with the entire chain or sentence. Examples of appropriate questions are included in Chapter 3 under "How to Establish Specific Language Structures."

Also, probe for instances of morphological constructions, such as plurals and past tenses in untrained words. These are critical examples of similar task generalization. For instance, when a student has been taught that she adds the /s/ sound when she sees two or more cats as opposed to just one cat, you want to determine if she can use her grammar in a generative fashion by saying words such as *cups, cats,* and *rakes* in response to two or more of those items the first time she encounters them.

Generalization Training

If through the probing you find that the student has failed to generalize, select at least one or two other people who will give the student the communication and language training prescribed by the initial instructor in at least one or two different settings. The only difference between this training and the training given by the initial instructor is the number of trials required and the amount of time involved. Only three or four trials on each specified task should be required. These can be presented during physical therapy, on a shopping trip, while learning to match socks, at lunchtime, while watching TV, or wherever it is agreeable for the person(s) selected to do the generalization training.

The communication and langauge instructor ideally should provide the generalization probing and training cards and a clipboard so that the person who is doing the generalization training has information which specifies exactly what he should show the student and what he should say to him. In addition, these cards contain a space for the reinforcement schedule and space to record the student's responses as either correct or incorrect. A clipboard is easy to carry around and makes it possible to attach pictures or other materials used in the initial instruction and the generalization training and probing card so that responses can be recorded immediately regardless of where the probing occurs. No prompting or reinforcing should occur during *probing.* However, during generalization *training,* the same reinforcing and prompting procedures the communication and language instructor is using would be appropriate. Therefore, it would be possible to use the same recording procedures on the generalization probing and training cards as are used on the data recording sheets, including prompted correct and prompted incorrect responses.

Ideally, these cards should be returned to the communication and langauge instructor daily. Then she can be responsible for graphing the data and determining when criterion is reached, etc. Essentially, the person doing the probing should have his responsibilities simplified as much as possible. Remember that you are asking another person, who is also a very busy person, to assume an added responsibility.

When the data reveal that criterion is met with at least one generalization trainer in at least one setting as determined by the communication and language instructor, probing identical to that described above must be done again to determine whether the student has now generalized to settings, people, antecedent stimuli, and tasks where he has never received specific language training. If he has not done so, the procedure must be repeated, adding new trainers and new settings until he does generalize to nontrained settings with people who have never participated in any training (Murdock, Garcia, & Hardman, 1977).

We suggest that you can train severely language impaired individuals to generalize appropriately to similar language tasks by providing them with abundant learning opportunities. Overlearning is perhaps the most obvious approach to this problem. While normal individuals may need only a few experiences with adding the /s/ or /z/ sound to communicate that they are talking about more than one of something, language handicapped students may need to use that plural construction many, many times before they will generalize correctly to express a plural on which they have not received specific training. The important thing for communication and language instructors is to realize this and plan their programs to systematically incorporate training for particular morphological and syntactic forms until appropriate generalization occurs. The student will not have the language of a normal $3^{1}/_{2}$- or 4-year-old student until he has mastered this kind of generalization.

In summary, when prompting is no longer necessary and you have thinned the reinforcement schedule to VR 5 or even less in your regular training sessions, you will begin probing for generalization. If the probing indicates that the communication and language behaviors the student has learned with you are not generalizing to other people, other settings, different discriminative stimuli, and similar communication and language tasks, begin the generalization training.

In your regular training sessions, use the tasks frequently as review tasks that you interject whenever a student is not experiencing a lot of success on a new task she is learning. This procedure not only guarantees that the student gets ample opportunity to review, but it also guarantees that she will experience a high level of success and reinforcement during communication and language instruction.

CHAPTER 6

SERVICE DELIVERY MODEL

JANE Y. MURDOCK

THERE are three points made thus far in CLIP that are basic to its successful implementation. First, communication and language instruction with moderately to severely communicatively impaired students should occur in at least three major environments: home, school, and community. Second, communication and language instruction for this population should be continuous throughout the waking hours, not just two or three times weekly or once daily for 20 minutes or half an hour. Third, everyone who comes into regular contact with these students should have some knowledge of: (1) already mastered communication and language skills so that they can be introduced naturally and frequently and the students can be reinforced by communicating successfully, (2) communication and language skills that the students are presently working on and what correction procedures and reinforcing consequences are being used in order to accelerate mastery, and (3) communication and language skills that are not currently expected so that they will not be presented because this is almost guaranteeing that the student will fail. Meeting these criteria greatly enhances the probability that moderately to severely communicatively impaired individuals will both learn and generalize their communicative skills (Carr, 1980; Carr & Kologinsky, 1983; Cavallaro, 1983; Hart & Risley, 1975; Hart & Risley, 1980; Hart & Rogers-Warren, 1978; Koegel & Rincover, 1974; Kopchick & Lloyd, 1976; McGee, Krantz, Mason, & McClannahan, 1983; Nietupski, Scheutz, & Ockwood, 1980; Rogers-Warren & Warren, 1980).

However, communication and language intervention with moderately to severely communicatively impaired populations traditionally has been on a one-to-one basis in an isolated area. Furthermore, it has been episodic, in that the language instructor removes individually selected students that he or she is working with from the classroom or other natural setting for a fixed period of time on a daily, semiweekly, or weekly basis (Hart & Risley, 1980; Hart & Rogers-Warren, 1978; Kopchick & Lloyd, 1976; Nietupski et al., 1980; Rogers-Warren & Warren, 1980). Considering the implications of these training procedures for a typical speech-language pathologist, he or she could deliver services to a maximum of 55 students a week, assuming that each student is seen once weekly. If students were seen daily, the case load could not be more than 11. These figures were arrived at by dividing a 9:00 A.M. to 3:30 P.M. academic day into half-hour segments with an hour for lunch and no other commitments on the part of the speech-language pathologist, such as testing, report writing, staffings, in-service trainings, or other meetings. These figures also assume that not more than a total of 30 minutes is devoted to each student, including locating the student and getting to and from the isolated therapy setting. They further assume that there is no interaction between the speech-language pathologist and classroom teachers, parents, or others in the student's environment outside of the therapy situation.

In reality, these time guidelines simply are not feasible. Speech-language pathologists normally have extensive testing, staffing, and meeting schedules. They also spend considerable time consulting with teachers, parents, and administrators. Furthermore, they normally are required to provide in-service training for teachers and paraprofessionals, usually on a weekly basis on Friday afternoons. In addition, they conduct periodic workshops for parents and other interested individuals.

Considering these realities, a very efficient speech-language pathologist may be able to deliver episodic services on a one-to-one basis to a maximum of 20 students, actually instructing each of them two or three times a week for approximately 20 minutes each session. In academic or clinical settings that provide communication and language instruction for moderately to severely handicapped students, the vast majority of the students need and are legally entitled to receive that instruction.

In addition to severely limiting the number of students who can receive instruction, there are other inherent problems in the traditional service delivery model. One of the most serious is the failure on the part of the students to generalize the communication and language skills they have mastered with an individual who presented carefully controlled discriminative stimuli in an isolated setting to other people in other environments or to other tasks (Brookshire, 1967; Carr, 1980; Carr & Kologinsky, 1983; Cavallaro, 1983; Engel, Brandriet, Erickson, Gronhovd, & Gunderson, 1966; Johnston & Johnston, 1972; McGee et al., 1983; Mulac & Tomlinson, 1977; Murdock, Garcia, & Hardman, 1977; Nietupski et al., 1980; Schuler, 1980). Furthermore, teachers, parents, and others who have a great deal of contact with the student are usually only partially aware of the communication and language skills the student has mastered, skills he is currently working on, and skills that are not presently in his repertoire.

They are usually even less knowledgeable about how the speech-language pathologist or other instructor teaches him: What discriminative stimuli are presented to signal the student to respond and how these should be varied, what reinforcers are delivered following correct responses and how these should be varied and thinned, or what correction or prompting procedures are used following incorrect responses and how these should be gradually faded. Consequently, individuals who interact with the student on a continuous basis at school, at home, or in the community are not able to extend the communication and language instruction the student is receiving from the individual instructor into natural environments where, eventually, naturally occurring cues and consequences will signal and reinforce the student throughout his waking hours.

INCIDENTAL TEACHING AND/OR MILIEU INSTRUCTION

In order to accomplish more efficient acquisition and generalization, several instructional models have been developed which emphasize teaching in natural environments. Some of them also emphasize group rather than individual instruction. One of the first was developed by Koegel and Rincover (1974). They investigated teaching eight autistic students in a classroom environment after discovering that the attending, imitating, and speaking skills the students had mastered in a one-to-one instructional arrangement did not generalize to the classroom or even to a group of two children and one teacher. Furthermore, the students did not acquire new behaviors appropriate to classroom learning. Consequently, the one-to-one instructional procedures gradually were phased into the classroom situation. This was very successful, in that the students learned to respond appropriately with verbal and nonverbal behaviors that they had previously learned but failed to exhibit in the classroom, and, in addition, they learned other behaviors, such as telling time, printing letters, and solving basic arithmetic problems in a classroom situation with one teacher and eight students.

Kopchick and Lloyd (1976) presented a total communication model for the severely language impaired. Their definition of total communication went beyond the traditional definition of using all available language modes for communication to incorporating such a program into a communicatively impaired individual's total environment on a twenty-four-hour basis. Their rationale for this was that language must be functional, that is, it must be used to manipulate and modify one's environment. Therefore, a total communication program should operate where one's physical and personal needs can be met in order to enhance possibilities of reinforcement and generalization.

Hart and Risley (1974, 1975) investigated the effects of incidental teaching on the language acquisition of disadvantaged preschoolers. Incidental teaching involved responding to a communication initiated by a child with focused attention or focused attention plus a verbal cue. If the child did not respond to the cue, then the instructor would prompt the child by requesting the terminal behavior, providing a partial prompt of the terminal behavior, or providing a complete model of the terminal behavior. While these instructional techniques were actually on a one-to-one basis since the adult responded to each individually initiated communication, the instruction occurred in settings where natural cues and consequences were available. Hart and Risley found that specific instruction and continual prompts were not necessary for the children to learn to generate and maintain a variety of language behaviors. Furthermore, the language readily generalized to people who had not participated in the instruction. Hart and Risley (1980) re-examined the children involved in their earlier experiments and compared their language usage to other disadvantaged children and to middle-class children of college parents. They found that language usage and language elaboration of the experimental group of disadvantaged children shifted from a pattern similar to the disadvantaged control group to a pattern similar to the middle-class children.

Hart and Rogers-Warren (1978) presented a milieu teaching model as a bridge between the training environment and the actual talking environment. The training environment was a traditional one-to-one situation, which was very effective for producing discrete verbal responses. However, in addition to being very expensive, such discrete trial learning did not generalize to other settings and other persons. In other words, the children had learned the form of the language, but they had not learned how to make it function for them. In an attempt to ensure functional usage, the technology used in the training environment was integrated with a technology of teaching talking. Talking environments differ in many important ways from environments designed to teach language behaviors. One of the obvious differences is the expense involved. But more importantly, the talking environment includes a variety of people and a multiplicity of stimuli, and the language used is varied in form and purpose. Although models for appropriate language occur in the talking environment, children may or may not attend to them. Hart and Rogers-Warren felt that the effectiveness of the talking environment may lie, in part, on this very haphazard nature of it, particularly for normal children. However, if language acquisition doesn't occur as anticipated in the talking environment, the language-impaired child simply fails to learn. Thus, they developed the milieu teaching model to integrate the teaching and talking environments.

Milieu teaching occurs in the environment where the child spends the majority of his or her time — at home, at school, or in the ward where he or she might live. All of the normal activities a child encounters are potentially available as occasions for teaching language. However, the child's communicative skills are assessed carefully in the milieu setting as are the stimuli that evoke and reinforce or punish language. Language skills are taught sequentially on the basis of individual abilities. Regardless of the level of a child's language skills, adults in the environment focus on making the child's language functional by responding to it with their attention and providing the objects or services the child requested. In addition to assessing a child's present language skills, the milieu model requires arranging the environment to prompt the use of language and training adults to ensure that the child's language functions for him or her.

Rogers-Warren and Warren (1980) modified the Hart and Risley (1974, 1975) incidental teaching technique in order to use it with one moderately and two severely language-impaired children because these children did not initiate communicative interactions, which was necessary before any incidental teaching could occur with Hart and Risley's disadvantaged preschoolers. Rogers-Warren and Warren trained classroom teachers to ask a child to verbally request or describe a variety of available materials whenever the child approached a particular item. The teachers were further trained in how to prompt and reinforce the children. In addition, the teachers were made aware of the different criteria for appropriate verbal reponses for each child. These procedures resulted in greatly increasing the amount of language displayed by the language-impaired children in the classroom environment.

McGee, Krantz, Mason, and McClannahan (1983) also modified Hart and Risley's incidental teaching procedures in order to establish communicative behaviors and promote generalization of those behaviors with autistic youth in a community-based program. Language instruction took place in natural settings while simultaneously teaching other necessary home-living skills.

Nietupski, Scheutz, and Ockwood (1980) examined communication therapy services for severely handicapped students and concluded that the isolated therapy model was not the most efficient model. They presented a five-step plan to implement an integrated therapy model alternative that would provide communication training in natural environments throughout the school day in which the therapist and teacher would cooperatively teach communication and language skills *in the classroom.* At each successive step, the teacher would assume more direct responsibility for delivering language instruction.

Cavallaro (1983) also noted the acquisition and generalization advantages for handicapped students of language intervention in natural settings. She provided some rules of thumb for incidental teaching or milieu models. These included: (1) using many opportunities to teach language, (2) prompting systematically, (3) using concise language and waiting for the student to respond, (4) using materials and assistance to reinforce language, and (5) keeping interactions brief and pleasant.

While there may be some differences in the above models regarding whether to deliver communication and language instruction on an individual or a group basis, there is no disagreement about delivering instruction in natural environments. Considering the expense involved in one-to-one instruction and the limiting effect it has on the number of students who can receive communication and language instruction, group instruction in natural environments appears to be a highly desirable service delivery model. Furthermore, group instruction makes it possible to use a peer as a model and to reinforce one student's appropriate attending and responding with descriptive praise, using it as a model for other students to imitate. The real lagniappe of group instruction may very well lie in the fact that each student in the group becomes sensitized to the others' communicative styles and abilities, as well as learning to imitate the instructor's reinforcing behaviors. Ideally, such a model would incorporate systematic training and supervision of individuals who interact with moderately to severely communicatively impaired students throughout their waking hours.

CLIP'S SERVICE DELIVERY MODEL

According to Hart and Rogers-Warren (1978), there are three major components of a milieu teaching model. These are: (1) arrange the environment, (2) assess the communication and language skills, and (3) train others who interact with the communicatively impaired individual on a regular basis in natural environments. In addition, arrangements must be made to ensure that overall group objectives are implemented so that the *group* instruction is not, in fact, *individual* instruction that happens to be delivered while other students are present. Consideration must be given also to group size and suggestions for holding students' attention that are particularly applicable when instructing a group of students. Finally, the implications for reaching more communicatively impaired individuals will be discussed.

Arranging the Environment

Ensure that there are many appealing objects and activities available. Students are not likely to ask for things that they do not want. Use all naturally occurring events as occasions to teach communicative behaviors. It is extremely desirable to teach vocabulary, requesting, rejecting, and commenting behaviors related to eating, toileting, dressing, grooming, cooking, swinging, walking, washing dishes, doing arithmetic, buying groceries, repairing machinery, doing laundry, etc., while engaging in those activities and learning related behaviors.

In many instances, the environments are already arranged. They simply need to be used advantageously. In some instances, special modifications will be necessary, such as providing more desirable objects and activities and ensuring that naturally occurring reinforcers only reinforce appropriate behaviors as was noted in Chapter 3. Special physical arrangements may be necessary when instructing students who are severely impaired or students who are new to the situation. Review arrangements for working with individual students which are described at the beginning of Chapter 3. When individual instruction is necessary, keep it within the natural environment as much as possible and have someone who is with the student on a regular basis coteaching with you from the beginning.

Assessment

Component 2, assessment, was accomplished through taking the spontaneous communication and language samples and analyzing them using Tables 2-1, 2-2, and 2-3. These records also apprised you of individuals who interact regularly with the student and how they respond to her communicative attempts. You also have had an opportunity to observe at least three major environments to determine whether materials and activities are available that the student wants so that they can serve as discriminative stimuli to evoke the communicative responses and as natural reinforcers for those responses.

Training Others

Your role as a speech-language pathologist or other qualified communication and language specialist becomes one of training others to deliver instruction on a regular basis throughout the students' waking hours. The following example presents an instructional training model that can be used to train classroom teachers and others to deliver communication and language instruction to a small group of students. It includes a recommended schedule that provides for direct services to several small groups of students, while at the same time providing for on-site in-service training for teachers and other professionals, paraprofessionals, parents, or anyone who is interested and available. The instructional setting in the following example is the classroom. Ms. Maria Garcia is the speech-language pathologist and Mr. Tom Adams is the classroom teacher.

Model for Training Communication and Language Instructors

Sessions 1 and 2. Ms. Garcia is totally in charge. She presents all of the discriminative stimuli and correction procedures and delivers most of the reinforcers. Mr. Adams is present and observes and delivers some of the reinforcers.

Sessions 3 and 4. Ms. Garcia presents all of the discriminative stimuli and correction procedures. Both Ms. Garcia and Mr. Adams socially reinforce correct responses. However, if tangible reinforcers are being used, only Mr. Adams delivers them.

Sessions 5 and 6. Ms. Garcia and Mr. Adams present discriminative stimuli and correction procedures equally. Social reinforcers are delivered by both of them. However, only Mr. Adams delivers tangible reinforcers. If Mr. Adams presents discriminative stimuli incorrectly, fails to reinforce a correct response, or fails to correct or inadvertently reinforces an incorrect response, Ms. Garcia immediately takes over and models the appropriate teaching procedures, including delivering any tangible reinforcers.

Sessions 7 and 8. Mr. Adams takes over, presenting all of the discriminative stimuli and correction procedures and delivering all of the social and tangible reinforcers. Ms. Garcia only participates in delivering social reinforcers. However, if Mr. Adams presents discriminative stimuli incorrectly, fails to reinforce a correct response, or fails to correct or inadvertently reinforces an incorrect response, Ms. Garcia takes over and models correct teaching procedures, including delivering any tangible reinforcers.

Sessions 9 and 10. The instructional roles of Mr. Adams and Ms. Garcia are identical to those in sessions 7 and 8. However, ideally, a third instructor, such as a parent or a paraprofessional, joins the instructional situation. This individual will observe the teaching procedures as Mr. Adams did in sessions 1 and 2, and the entire cycle can be repeated with Mr. Adams providing the on-site in-service training.

After session 10, Ms. Garcia arranges her schedule so that she randomly observes Mr. Adams at least weekly during his communication and language instruction sessions. She provides feedback to him either orally or in writing following each observation. This feedback must recognize and appreciate good or excellent instructional behaviors as well as provide corrective feedback on mediocre or poor instructional procedures. The following is an example of a short note which Ms. Garcia might write to Mr. Adams:

> Congratulations, Tom! Your session today was great. Did you notice how Angelo's face lit up when he finally got the pants, shoes, and socks in the right sequence? And the way you brought Peter back into the action by reinforcing Nick was beautiful. If Carla spaces out on you again, you might try the same procedure with her. Also, try moving to a stronger prompt whenever a student fails to respond correctly after being prompted once. If they miss the second prompt, present a review task so that they can succeed and be reinforced. See you next week. Let me know if you need anything.
>
> Maria

This note combines sincere appreciation with constructive suggestions about how to correct problems and otherwise improve the instructional procedures. The attitudes reflected are attitudes that greatly enhance the probability that speech-language pathologists, behaviorists, and special educators will be able to work effectively with other professionals, paraprofessionals, and parents.

It may be necessary to create a situation that desensitizes extremely sensitive individuals who find it difficult to respond positively to even the most constructive and well-intentioned criticism. If so, set up an instructional session in which you deliberately make at least two or three instructional errors. Have several observers, including the very sensitive individuals, present or have the session videotaped. The observers are expected to be able to identify the errors and provide corrective feedback.

In actual practice, I have found that enough instructional errors occur *unintentionally* and I do not have to make deliberate mistakes. Therefore, this procedure sets the tone that there is no such thing as a perfect instructor, whether he's a master speech-language pathologist, she's a super behaviorist, or he's a very special educator! All instructors make mistakes, particularly during the heat of a rapidly moving group instructional session with three to five students, at least two of whom are hyperactive. The important thing is to have someone around who can help correct those mistakes because it is an assigned part of their professional responsibilities. Therefore, their time is arranged so that they can observe instructional sessions and provide objective, constructive feedback.

While following this model may change the role of the speech-language pathologist quite dramatically, it has the advantage of providing communication and language instruction directly or indirectly to many more moderately or severely communicatively impaired students while at the same time providing continuous in-service training to teachers, other professionals, paraprofessionals, and parents.

Arranging Group and Individual Objectives in Natural Settings

There are major communication and language objectives that are relevant for all students at all times, such as: (1) expanding receptive and expressive vocabularies, (2) following instructions, (3) making requests, (4) interacting socially with greetings and other polite language, (5) describing things, (6) rejecting things, (7) commenting on other's communications, activities, objects, etc., and (8) using communicative forms to control behavior of self and others. It is necessary to keep these overall group objectives in mind. Consequently, "VIRSDRCC" is printed at the top of the data recording sheets. These letters stand for key words in each of the major group objectives: *vocabulary, intructions, requests, socially, describing, rejecting, commenting,* and *control.* Individual objectives will change constantly and will need to be specified. For example, Mr. Adams is showing Angelo, Carla, and Peter how to do their laundry. Within this milieu, he has the following group and individual communication and language objectives:

Group Objectives: VIRSDRCC related to laundromat.

Angelo's Objectives: (1) Select and count two quarters from a coin purse that contains at least three quarters, three dimes, three nickles, and three pennies. (2) Follow instructions to put large pieces of laundry, small pieces of laundry, and detergent in washer and coins in coin slot in that sequence. (3) Repeat the sequence aloud as a self-prompt if necessary. (4) Say "hello," "goodbye," and "thank you" or "please" to the attendant. (5) Use this same social language with anyone else in the laundromat who responds to him in a similar fashion.

Carla's Objectives: (1) Make eye contact and smile if attendant greets her. (2) Match and fold socks. (3) Request help by first touching to get attention and then gesturing.

Peter's Objectives: (1) Describe sheets as "big" and pillow cases as "little" in response to the question, "Is this big or little?" (2) Follow any two instructions in sequence, e.g., "Put the big sheets in the washer. Then put the little pillow cases in the washer." (3) If Carla shoves him, knocks his detergent over, kicks over his clothes basket, or otherwise engages in aggressive behaviors directed toward him, he is to tell Carla "Stop it!" loud enough for the instructor to hear.

Within this milieu, any communicative behaviors exhibited that are appropriate to the situation should be followed with attention, conversation, responding to the request, or any other natural consequences. The purpose of specifying overall group objectives is to ensure that instructors will keep them in mind and remember to provide opportunities for such responses and to reinforce them generously when they occur. Therefore, it may be necessary for some instructors to write them out completely when first using CLIP until they become automatic.

Attending to such overall group objectives is even more important for the communication and language instructor who is working in a more structured setting (e.g., the period during the school day that is identified as "Communication Training" or "Language Instruction"). *Group* instruction must include continuous involvement and objectives for the entire group, not brief periods of *individual* instruction that happens to occur while other students are present and waiting for their turn. In addition to continuously involving all of the students by reinforcing them for making responses related to the group objectives, specific procedures for involving the entire group are described in the following section on "Group Size and Suggestions for Holding Attention."

Group Size and Suggestions for Holding Attention

An ideal group size for severely communicatively impaired students is three to five. For less severely impaired students, a group of five is ideal, and seven is very manageable. In actual practice, I have worked with groups as large as 12, but this can be done only after working with students in smaller groups for some time so that you have become a discriminative stimulus for appropriate attending and responding behaviors.

The absolute limit for a structured, sit-down communication and language session is determined by the number of students you can have within your *reach.* This is important for two reasons: (1) so that you can deliver social reinforcers, such as shaking hands, patting, stroking, or tangible reinforcers, and (2) so that you can touch the student at the opposite physical location of any student you are providing with corrective feedback or otherwise working with individually. This touching the student who is the most removed from the individual student encloses the group and keeps all of the students attending. Also, keep your body oriented toward the entire group or even slightly toward the student you are touching. Turning your back on students excludes them from the ongoing activities.

When you are planning to request an individual to respond rather than the entire group, do not say that individual's name until the end of the statement or question that signals it is time for someone to respond. You might say, "I'm going to touch something. When I do, I want you to tell me or show me what we do with it. Ready (move your hand deliberately over several tools, finally touching one of them), what do we do with this, (pause) Beatrice?" As was noted in the attending section in Chapter 3, saying a student's name at the beginning is often a signal to all of the other students that they do not have to attend because they will not be asked to respond.

Another procedure that keeps all of the students in a group attending is to have all of them involved in determining whether an individual response is correct or not. Make the statement, "Listen (or watch) to see if this answer is right, (pause) everybody. Which of these do we use to brush our teeth with, (pause) Kenneth?" (Paused before "everybody" as well as "Kenneth" because this procedure can be used to let just one student "help" you.) If Kenneth selected the toothbrush, the students participate in the verbal praise and even applaud. If Kenneth is wrong, one of them can be selected to model or otherwise prompt the correct response.

Implications for Teaching More Communicatively Impaired Individuals

Table 6-1 is an example of a speech-language pathologist's schedule about five weeks after he implemented this service delivery model. He is observing each of seven small group sessions at least once a week on a random basis. He worked directly with each of these seven groups for at least two weeks while training the individuals he is now observing. Up to this point in time, he has consistently instructed three or four small groups per week on a daily basis. The schedule is divided into 30-minute time periods, with sessions lasting 20

TABLE 6-1

SAMPLE WEEKLY WORK SCHEDULE

	M	T	W	Th	F
8:30	Meetings and/or Planning	→	→	→	→
9:00	Sm. Grp. #8	→	→	→	→
9:30	Observe Grp. #3	Observe Grp. #1	Observe Grp. #7	Testing	Testing
10:00	Sm. Grp. #9	→	→	→	→
10:30	Indiv. Therapy	→	→	→	→
11:00	Sm. Grp. #10	→	→	→	→
11:30	Indiv. Therapy	→	→	→	→
12:00	Lunch	→	→	→	→
12:30	Sm. Grp. #11	→	→	→	→
1:00	Observe Grp. #6	Observe Grp. #4	Observe Grp. #2	Observe Grp. #5	Flexible Time
1:30	Indiv. Therapy	→	→	→	Flexible Time
2:00	Flexible time for feedback, individual therapy, consulting, staffing, testing, meetings, workshops, etc.				

minutes and 10 minutes left to interact with the instructor(s) and students and move to the next assignment.

This model provides for all group instruction to be completed by early afternoon. The 12:30 P.M. session is arranged especially to take place while the students eat lunch. While the observations are scheduled for 20 minutes, we have found that, normally, 10 minutes is adequate, and the remaining time can be used to provide feedback by writing notes to the instructor, such as the note Maria wrote to Tom, or jotting down notes to yourself to be discussed with the instructor at a later time.

While the schedule is tight between 9:00 A.M. and 2:00 P.M., there is a half hour for getting organized in the morning, a half hour for lunch, and from 2:00 P.M. on the time is flexible, providing time for feedback to other instructors, additional individual therapy, testing, consulting, staffing, meetings, workshops, etc. In practice, this plan provides for more flexible time than most schedules while, at the same time, providing for more direct and indirect services to communicatively impaired students.

The speech-language pathologist delivers direct services daily to a minimum of 19 students if there is an average of four students in each group and three students seen individually. He delivers indirect services to approximately 28 students. These figures do not include students whom he tests. Furthermore, the figures increase dramatically as the speech-language pathologist moves forward and continues to train individuals, including parents and paraprofessionals, until eventually he primarily observes group sessions on a weekly basis and only provides direct services on an individual basis until someone else is trained to provide those services. Considering that four time slots on this schedule are devoted to small groups of students who are seen daily, the speech pathologist conceivably could have a total of 27 time slots available to observe small groups on a weekly basis. Thus, a single speech-language pathologist could provide the programming and supervision for 88 students working in small groups with other instructors and still work with three individual students who are new to the program or too severely involved to benefit from group instruction.

In this model, individual therapy must also involve one other instructor and must take place in as natural an environment as possible, as was described at the beginning of Chapter 3. The co-instructor is one who is already instructing a small group of students in that setting so that members of her group can be brought into the instructional situation gradually until nearly all students are receiving small-group instruction in natural settings. Normally, only new students or those with severe multiple handicaps will receive individual instruction from the speech-language pathologist. Furthermore, for students with severe multiple handicaps, the speech-language pathologist's role will be one of training others to deliver direct communication and language services on a daily basis with regular supervision and programming provided by him.

Summary

In summary, this model provides for communication and language instruction in natural environments. The instruction can be continuous throughout the waking hours because the individuals delivering the instruction are those who are continuously with the students. Therefore, they know what skills each student has mastered, what skills are currently being worked on, and what skills are not currently in a student's repertoire. Furthermore, everyone who is normally present in natural environments, including teachers, paraprofessionals, volunteers, peers, parents, siblings, or great aunts, can be directly or indirectly involved in providing natural cues and consequences for the handicapped student's communication and language behaviors. This is highly desirable, not only because it minimizes the generalization problems experienced by the moderately to severely communicatively impaired population, but there is also good evidence that such natural contextual cues are important variables in the acquisition of communicative skills.

CHAPTER 7

ALTERNATIVE COMMUNICATION FORMS

JANE Y. MURDOCK

THERE are individuals who for a variety of known and unknown reasons cannot or do not speak. Many of them do not understand speech. Listening-speaking or auditory-vocal communication is highly desirable because it is the dominant mode in all cultures and it is the most flexible, varied, and semantically complete language system available (Schiefelbusch & Hollis, 1980). Nevertheless, it is only one form of communication. Just as we cannot insist that the deaf person "hear," we cannot insist that the nonspeaking person "speak." Placing each individual's needs first, it is essential to provide whatever viable form of communication that is available. This may be an alternative or augmentative technique. Throughout this chapter, the term *alternative* will be used to simplify the discourse. This is not to assume that speaking is excluded. An alternative or augmentative communication form is one which enhances communication by complementing whatever communicative skills, including vocal skills, an individual may possess. For some communicatively impaired individuals, this will be as sophisticated as writing their every need, desire, and idea. For some, it will be pairing communicative gestures with some vocalizations. For others, using simple gestures to express basic needs and desires may be the ultimate goal.

WHO NEEDS ALTERNATIVE COMMUNICATION FORMS?

Some words of caution, however, are in order. Avoid teaching signing or symbol systems just because they are the "in" thing to do. On the other hand, since speaking is the most desirable form of expressive communication, many parents, teachers, and others have unwarranted misgivings about teaching nonspeech communication systems. They fear that speech production will not be necessary and, thus, will be inhibited. This is highly unlikely. In fact, there is some evidence to the contrary that nonspeech systems may facilitate speech (Bricker & Bricker, 1974; Hodges & Deich, 1979; Kent, 1974; McDonald & Schulz, 1973; McNaughton & Kates, 1980, Schaeffer, 1980; Schaeffer, Musil, Kollinzas, 1980). Unwisely postponing nonspeech techniques until all attempts to teach vocal verbalization have failed may lead to delayed communication development and feelings of failure for both students and instructors (Harris & Vanderheiden, 1980).

However, alternative forms are not to be taught randomly to communicatively impaired populations. I recently had the experience of observing a profoundly retarded, legally blind young man whose language program included teaching him to use manual communication sign language, which was described as "a somewhat standardized system of manual and gestural communication and finger spelling." In order for this particular student to receive the communication, the signs were made in his hand, in spite of the fact that, although he did not speak, he responded very well to spoken instructions and requests. The young man had been in the signing program for almost a year and had never expressed himself with a sign without being physically prompted through the entire sign.

Another unfortunate example of inappropriate teaching content relates to a bright-eyed, smiling 8-year-old boy who responded immediately and appropriately to verbal instructions and requests but who had never said a word. A young behaviorist was certain that with appropriate shaping procedures, this nonspeaking child could learn to talk. After eight months of rigorous training sessions several times daily, the boy could not consistently make an "mmm" sound and, of course, had still never said a word. This child probably would have learned to express himself well if he had been given an alternative communication form. As it was, an academic year was wasted and a child's self-concept may have been seriously damaged.

These examples are important for several reasons. First, you must give some consideration to the intellectual, physical, and sensory impairments that are present. Students must have regular auditory and visual acuity tests. They may not be speaking or responding to speech because they cannot hear well. They may not be signing or responding to signs because they cannot see well. Second, consideration must be given to the abstraction level of the communication form. Many signing systems involve visual symbols that are just as abstract as any spoken or written word and, in order to learn them, an individual must be able to symbolize (Dever, 1974; Moores, 1980; Schiefelbusch, 1974). Finally, you must be responsive to your students. If they are not learning what you are trying to teach them, *you,* not they, are at fault.

There are prerequisite behaviors for any form of communication. If your preprogram observations revealed a student who was involved with objects but not with people, who failed to make eye contact, who did not respond to your presence or the presence of others, who did not respond to the human voice, who did not smile or scowl, and who failed to use gestures to communicate basic needs and desires, she does not have the prerequisite skills for complex communication training (Uzirgis & Hunt, 1975). Instruction with this student must begin with establishing the function of communication before complex language and communication forms can be realized. She must learn that when she deliberately engages in certain communicative behaviors, such as pointing, showing, or handing, she is sending messages that will have generally predictable effects on those who receive them. Interested readers are referred to Sternberg, Battle, and Hill (1980) and Woolman (1980) for further information about prelanguage or presymbolic training.

Before making the determination that an alternative form of communication is appropriate, some determination about the student's ability to develop spoken language must be made and this can be tenuous at best (Shane, 1980). However, you have much information about the student's present communicative behaviors and potential for communication from the spontaneous communication and language samples and the receptive and expressive language tests. You know, for instance, how, or whether, the student is presently communicating. Does she talk, sign, use some symbol system, use a communication board, gesture paired with vocalization, or gesture without vocalizations?

According to Harris and Vanderheiden (1980), individuals may be nonvocal for a variety of reasons, each of which requires a different intervention program. Harris and Vanderheiden developed more inclusive descriptions of nonvocal individuals than simply calling them nonvocal, including nonvocal hearing impaired (NVHI), nonvocal mentally retarded (NVMR), nonvocal autistic (NVA), and nonvocal severely physically handicapped (NVSPH). A person who cannot hear usually has great difficulty imitating the spoken word. A severely mentally retarded student may be nonvocal because of cognitive deficits or symbolization difficulties. An autistic student may be nonvocal because of a failure to process auditory sensory input or a failure to symbolize, particularly symbols related to language. A cerebral palsied student with normal intelligence may be nonvocal because of impairment to the vocal musculature, respiration, and/or fine motor coordination needed for speech. The same nonspeech intervention technique would not be appropriate for all of these students. The first student's hearing impairment may be solely responsible for his failure to speak. If medical intervention and/or a hearing aid fail to correct the problem, a nonspeech visual communication system, probably manual signing, is definitely in order. The severely mentally retarded student, in all probability, would do no better learning to sign or write than she did learning to speak. However, she may do very well communicating with gestures. The autistic student might do very well in a total communication program or interacting with a microcomputer. The student with cerebral palsy, in all probability, could master the English alphabet and communicate very successfully using a typewriter adapted to her physical handicap. Furthermore, there is some evidence that all of them could benefit from technological advances discussed in Chapter 8, particularly those related to computer technology.

Initially, no instructor is going to pick the perfect intervention procedure for *every* communicatively impaired student that she contacts. Therefore, make the determination that it is better to err in the direction of thinking that a student is more capable than he actually is than to err in the other direction, in which case the student is not given an opportunity to learn as sophisticated a communication form as he is capable of learning. Keeping accurate data and responding to those data will preclude the possibility of keeping a student in any program that is beyond his intellectual, physical, or sensory capabilities for any extended period of time. Such responsive data recording and accountability procedures are covered in detail in Chapter 4.

The ability to imitate may be the best single predictor of how well a student will do in any communication training. Although there has been considerable controversy regarding imitation training and language development in recent years (Rees, 1975), communication programs that use imitation as the basis for initial language acquisition have been successful, particularly with moderately to severely communicatively impaired populations (Cole & Cole, 1981; Gray & Ryan, 1973; Guess, Sailor, & Baer, 1976; Hinerman, 1983; Kent, 1974; Lovaas, 1966; Murdock & Hartmann, 1975; Striefel, 1974). Furthermore, much of the controversy over imitation and language development may be because of different interpretations of what imitation is. These can range from verbatim repetition of a model immediately after it is presented, to partial mirroring of such aspects as length, order, complexity, or structure (Cole & Cole, 1981). Considering imitation in a broad sense, it is difficult to imagine that one would learn any language or communication system for which there was no model.

If a student can imitate sounds and words, the first efforts should be to teach him to talk. If he cannot imitate sounds and words but can imitate motor movements, an augmentative communication system such as manual communication is in order. If he cannot imitate sounds or motor movements because of severe motor involvement such as that experienced by many students with cerebral palsy but, nevertheless, smiles, tries to gain attention with vocalization, and obviously is attempting to communicate, then a communication board, one of the symbol systems, or a microcomputer may be the answer.

The remainder of this chapter presents some examples of communication forms that are augmentative or alternatives to the auditory-vocal form. It is not intended to be exhaustive or to cover any of them in great detail. To do so would take several volumes. It is intended to present the case for using alternative communication forms and to apprise the reader of some of the many alternatives available. In addition, the interested reader is referred to *Non-Speech Language Initiation Program* (Carrier & Peak, 1975), *Language Acquisition Program for the Retarded or Multiply Impaired* (Kent, 1974), *Communication Assessment and Intervention Strategies* (Lloyd, 1976), *Total Communication: A Signed Speech Program for Nonverbal Children* (Schaeffer, Musil, & Kollonzas, 1980), *Nonspeech Language and Communication: Analysis and Intervention* (Schiefelbusch, 1980), *Language Intervention from Ape to Child* (Schiefelbusch and Hollis, 1979) *Communication for the Speechless* (Silverman, 1982), *Handbook of Blissymbolics* (Silverman, McNaughton, & Kates, 1978), *Amer-Ind Gestural Code Based on Universal American Indian Hand Talk* (Skelley, 1979), and *Non-Vocal Communication Resource Book* (Vanderheiden & Grilley, 1976).

Language is a system of symbols. A word, whether spoken, written, signed, or represented with a plastic chip or a graphic symbol, is just a *symbol.* It is *not* the thing, or the action, or the relation between the thing or the action. Languages are made up of abstract symbols that are used to represent meaning.

VISUALLY PERMANENT SYMBOL SYSTEMS

This section is devoted to symbol systems that are alternatives to speaking or manual communication forms, in that they do not place the same strain on short-term memory that a spoken word or a manual sign does. A spoken word, a manual sign, and a gesture are gone instantaneously and cannot be referred to again except as the receiver can recall them. A written word, a plastic chip, a picture, or other permanent visual configurations can remain before an individual for an indeterminate length of time. This section begins with the most obvious permanent visual symbol system (i.e., the written form of the spoken communication) and concludes with pictographic and ideographic Bliss symbols.

Written Language

Communication boards are obvious forms of the written mode and have long been used by cerebral palsied students (Roe, 1948; Sayre, 1963). A communication board can be set up in many ways. The following example is an adaptation of the Fitzgerald Key (Fitzgerald, 1966). The words selected are only samples. A student's communication board should contain individualized, functional vocabulary.

Communication boards similar to Table 7-1 are frequently set up with numbers and the alphabet at the top or margins for students who can spell, in addition to recognizing whole printed words. Sometimes color codes are used as prompts. For instance, the red area on the board may contain only action words. For an excellent discussion of various communication boards as augmentative communication techniques, see McDonald (1980).

TABLE 7-1

COMMUNICATION BOARD ADAPTED FROM THE FITZGERALD KEY

	People	Action Words	Descriptive Words	What	Interests	Where
CORE	I, me	need	happy	food	TV	home
VOCABU-	Mom	want	sad	water	stereo	school
LARY	Daddy	eat	mad	toilet	toy	cupboard
	teacher	drink	more		puzzle	bathroom
		help				
	boy	work	hungry	clothes	radio	park
EXPANDED	girl	play	thirsty	bed	pencil	drugstore
VOCABU-	you	sleep	sick	chair	telephone	classroom
LARY	friend	draw	tired	table	paper	church
	sister	read	funny		animal	shop
	brother	write	good		number	restaurant
	doctor	love	hot			
	nurse	like	cold		*Additional Symbols & Manners*	
	therapist	wash	not		hello	
		come	tired		goodbye	
		see	afraid		please	
		hear			thank you	
		talk/speak			I'm sorry	
		smell			question	
		taste			opposite	
		go			same	
					different	

Be cautious making assumptions about communicatively impaired indiv-diuals. Do not assume that a student who cannot learn to talk cannot learn to read and write. Furthermore, do not assume that intellectual functioning below an IQ score of 50 means that an individual cannot learn to read or at least recognize written words well enough to provide some form of functional communication. Murdock (1978b) found that a 15-year-old, nonverbal female with an IQ of 32 could read printed words and phrases well enough to use them to express her needs and desires in much the same manner as one would use a communication board. However, printing the words and phrases on lightweight manila paper was thought to be more suitable than a communication board for a student who had excellent mobility. LaVigna (1977) established word-object association through the written word with autistic children who had previously displayed no special ability in spelling or reading words. Marshall and Hegrenes (1972) taught an autistic boy to read and type letters, words, and phrases. Using written language to communicate is very desirable because most of the population over the age of six or seven can understand the communication.

The disadvantages of the written forms described above are that they are cumbersome and rarely used outside of clinical or educational environments.

The ideal form of written communication is for the communicatively impaired individual to be able to write. With many of the moderately to severely communicatively impaired, there are perceptual, cognitive, and/or fine motor deficits present, also. Electric typewriters have, however, been adapted by placing a Plexiglas™ cover or some other device over the keyboard so that students with cerebral palsy and other motor impairments can locate and strike the target key without striking several adjacent keys because a ridge surrounding the key prevents the finger or pointer from slipping.

Other Permanent Visual Symbol Systems

This section presents nonspeech symbol systems which use symbols that vary in size, color, shape, or other attributes in order to provide an individual with the means of receiving and/or sending messages. Some of them are based on the work of David and Ann Premack (Premack, 1970, 1971; Premack & Premack, 1972, 1974). The symbols used are plastic chips of different geometric shapes that have no pictographic or ideographic relationship to the words they represent. One of the advantages of such a symbol system is that it does not require the short-term memory capability that a spoken word or a sign requires. The plastic chip is visually present for as long as it takes to process the message and formulate the response. Furthermore, the communicatively impaired student can use the symbols without having to produce them in the sense that they would have to produce a spoken word or a manual sign. Much of the early research using symbol systems was done with primates. However, Premack and Premack (1974) used the system to teach a nonverbal autistic boy with considerable success.

NONSLIP. Non-Speech Language Initiation Program, or NonSLIP, is a symbol system developed by Carrier and Peak and based on Premack and Premack's research (Carrier, 1974, 1976; Carrier & Peak, 1975). Each symbol has a unique shape and each is color coded for syntax (all nouns are one color, verbs another color, and so forth). Instead of speaking, writing, or identifying words and stringing them together to make sentences, the students select and arrange plastic chips in the proper sequence (e.g., article, noun, verb auxiliary, verb, preposition, article, noun). McLean and McLean (1978) reported using NonSLIP with some success with autistic children, and Carrier and Peak (1975) reported on its successful implementation with severely and profoundly retarded individuals.

A possible criticism of the program is that some of the language is not functional (e.g., *the cow is sitting on the car*) (Schuler & Baldwin, 1981). However, as Premack and Premack (1974) noted, the plastic chips can be used to represent anything you want them to represent. It's doubtful, for instance, that *cow* will be a highly relevant word for most students to learn. Therefore, it seems that chip could be changed to represent *milk* or whatever you want it to represent that is functional.

REBUS SYMBOLS. A rebus is an alternative communication form based on symbols that represent entire words or parts of words. Most of the forms are pictographic, that is, they are actual drawings of the words or syllables they represent or they can be drawings of another thing with the same name. For instance, a drawing of waves may represent *sea* and *see*. Common examples of rebuses are those used on road signs and in international airports.

Anyone can design rebus symbols. However, Clark, Davies, and Woodcock (1974) published a set that has become somewhat of a standard. It contains 818 different rebuses and over 1,200 combinations of rebuses with letters. There is also a *Peabody Rebus Reading Program* available which begins with a vocabulary of rebuses and gradually fades into traditional printed words (Woodcock, Clark, Davies, 1968).

Rebuses have been very useful in place of or combined with written words on communication boards (McDonald & Schultz, 1973; Vanderheiden & Harris-Vanderheiden, 1976). The communicative task is simplified by: (1) selecting a picture of the word that represents the idea or thought, rather than a more abstract written word or plastic chip, and (2) requiring only a pointing, looking, or touching response as opposed to the fine motor requirements of writing, typing, or manually signing (Hollis & Carrier, 1978).

BLISSYMBOLICS. Bliss symbols are primarily pictographic or ideographic in that the symbols represent a thing, an idea, or a concept. However, some Bliss symbols are necessarily arbitrary symbols and others are also quite abstract and require considerable ability to symbolize. Bliss (1965) developed the system as an international language, which he dreamed would be used in commerce, industry, and science and, eventually, might bring about world peace. It was first applied as an augmentative aid to speech with physically handicapped, nonspeaking children at the Ontario Crippled Children's Center in Toronto, Canada in 1971 (McNaughton & Kates, 1980) and was incorporated into communication boards by Vanderheiden in Wisconsin in 1976 (Hollis & Carrier, 1978). Blissymbolics is a semantically based system, in that most components relate directly or indirectly to meaning. Thus, the symbol for the pronoun *I* would not be the same as the body part *eye*, as it could be in other symbol systems.

There are four types of Blissymbolics: (1) pictographic, such as a line drawing of a *building, tree, man, woman,* etc., (2) ideographic, such as a drawing of a heart to represent *love*, the top half of a diamond which looks like a roof to represent *protection,* arrows pointing toward or away from a vertical line to represent *come* or *go*, etc., (3) arbitrary symbols, such as a question mark to represent *what,* a dot preceding a short slanted line to represent *that,* a dot following the same short slanted line to represent *this,* etc., and (4) mixed, in which pictographic, ideographic, and/or arbitrary components are combined

(McNaughton & Kates, 1980). Meaning can be determined by size, position, orientation, spacing, pointers, and positional reference of the symbols also. According to McDonald (1980), a relatively few symbols can be combined in a rather straightforward, simple system to represent thousands of meanings.

MANUAL COMMUNICATION SYSTEMS

Research studies with deaf children who also have deaf parents suggest that they are superior in academic achievement, social-emotional adjustment, reading, and the ability to express themselves in English when compared to their deaf peers who have hearing parents (Moores, 1980). Whether this is because of the early visual communicative behaviors the children learned from their deaf parents as opposed to being raised in a communicative environment which primarily depended upon auditory input and vocal output, or whether the empathy of the deaf parents for their child's deafness made the difference, cannot be determined. My own opinion is that empathy and love are not enough, but that language or some other viable form of communication is critical for academic success and social-emotional adjustment for *all* individuals. The data related to the deaf population, along with the Gardners' highly publicized use of American Sign Language as a way to investigate language potential in primates (Gardner & Gardner, 1969), lead to investigating the possibilities of trying manual communication systems with moderately to severely handicapped, nonspeaking individuals.

Sign Languages

Until 1971 the terms *manual communication* and *sign language* referred to various forms of signing systems used by deaf persons throughout the world. In 1971 and 1972, educational manual communication systems were developed that were based on English and American Sign Language (also referred to as Ameslan and ASL). While there is considerable overlapping between ASL and English, there are also distinct semantic and syntactic differences. For example, ASL has no articles and does not differentiate the pronouns *he, she,* and *it.* There are markers for past, present, future, and progressive verb tenses but without the redundancy present in English. Furthermore, while ASL usually follows a subject-predicate word order, the word order is relatively free under two conditions: If the verb is intransitive (does not act on an object) or if it is transitive (acts on an object) and the subject and object are nonreversible (Mayberry, 1976).

Consequently, primarily for educational purposes, signing systems have been developed in the United States which semantically and syntactically more closely parallel English. Seeing Essential English or SEE 1 (Anthony, 1971) borrows much of its lexicon from ASL. However, when the semantic boundaries of an English word differ from the sign, those of the sign are changed to conform to those of the English word. Each English pronoun and article has a SEE 1 sign. Verb tenses are similar to English verb tenses with signs for tense markers and auxiliary verbs. The greatest difference between ASL and SEE 1 is syntax (Mayberry, 1976).

Signing Exact English or SEE 2 (Gustason, Pfetzing, & Zowalkow, 1972) is very similar to SEE 1. Most of the vocabulary comes from ASL, and articles and pronouns are similar to SEE 1. SEE 2 follows English word order but has fewer tense markers and auxiliaries (e.g., is, are, was, were, etc.) than SEE 1 (Mayberry, 1976). According to Mayberry (1976), SEE 2 is best characterized as a limited version of SEE 1. Furthermore, ASL relies more heavily upon meaning than SEE 2, in that words that are pronounced the same but have different meanings are signed the same in SEE 2 but signed differently in ASL because the two words differ conceptually (Moores, 1980).

Signed English was developed at Gallaudet College for preschool deaf children (Bornstein, 1973, 1974). The vocabulary is identical to ASL. It has pronouns and articles similar to SEE 1 and SEE 2, limited tense markers and auxiliary verbs, and the word order follows English (Mayberry, 1976). Schaeffer, Musil, and Kollinzas (1980) recommend using a system they refer to as Signed English which, according to them, mirrors spoken English and is based on SEE 2 and *The Signed English Dictionary* by Bornstein, Hamilton, Saulnier, and Roy (1975).

According to Mayberry (1976), the new system that differs most from ASL is Linguistics of Visual English or LOVE (Wampler, 1971). Love uses pronouns, articles, tense markers, auxiliaries, and follows English word order. However, LOVE differs more from ASL than SEE 1 and SEE 2 because LOVE is more phonemically than syntactically based. That is, it is based more upon the sound structure than the word order.

Other terms, such as *signed English, manual English, visual English* and *siglish* are used interchangeably to refer to the use of ASL in English word order with or without additional signs for pronouns, articles, verb tenses, and auxiliary verbs. Usually, such English signing is a potpourri of signs from all of the systems, resulting in pidgin ASL English (Mayberry, 1976).

Mayberry (1976) demonstrates the relationship between the newer systems to ASL and English by placing them on a syntactic and semantic continuum. On that continuum, SEE 1 is closer to English, signed English is closer to ASL, and SEE 2 is in the middle. She did not include LOVE with its phonemic emphasis on this syntactic and semantic continuum. Also, most of the signing systems involve some fingerspelling, which is literally signing each letter of the communication, and require that the user be able to spell.

It is obvious that the manual signing system selected for moderately to severely communicatively impaired individuals is critical. However, in both published research and individual education plans, it is rare that any precise description of the signing system used is given, which leaves the would-be signing instructor somewhat at a loss. According to a national survey of speech, hearing, and language services for the retarded (Fristoe, 1975), a large proportion of the respondents who were using signing systems used vocabulary from American Sign Language. According to Moores (1980), in manual communication programs with the severely handicapped, signs per se may not be used at all because it is unrealistic to assume that students with severe cognitive, physical, or emotional handicaps would benefit from manual communication systems as sophisticated as American Sign Language or one of its variants.

Nevertheless, there is considerable literature related to using signing successfully with autistic populations (Carr, 1979; Carr, Binkoff, Kologinsky, & Eddy, 1978; Carr, & Kologinsky, 1983; Fulwiler & Fouts, 1976; Remington & Clark, 1983; Schaeffer, 1978) and with other moderately to severely handicapped, nonspeaking populations (Duker & Morsink, 1984; Faw, Reid, Schepis, Fitzgerald, & Welty, 1981; Kent, 1974; Kopchick & Lloyd, 1976; Kopchick, Rombach, & Smilovitz, 1975).

Amer-Ind

Amer-Ind is a visual-motor communication system made up of gestures which are based on the hand talk of North American Indians (Skelley, 1979). It consists of 250 simple and, for the most part, immediately recognizable gestures, which can be combined to convey at least 2,500 words of any modern language. However, the gestures are based on concepts, not on words, and there are no required grammatical or structural rules. The gestures are also based on common, concrete human actions, such as curling your fingers toward your thumb as though holding a glass, raising your hand to parted lips, and tilting your head back slightly. Facial expressions add to the communicative effort. For example, hands are extended toward the front of the body with fingers tightly laced and tensed. The tensed hands are directed toward a person from whom help or assistance is sought. A distressed facial expression enhances the communication.

Amer-Ind has been useful with a variety of moderately to severely communicatively impaired, nonspeaking populations (Daniloff & Shafer, 1981; Roane, 1983; Silverman, 1980; Skelley, Schinsky, Smith, Donaldson, & Griffin, 1975; Skelley, Schinsky, Smith, & Fust, 1974). Unlike other visual-motor communication systems, Amer-Ind has no grammar and the gestures are very concrete. Most sign languages are symbolic, and the signs are as arbitrarily selected as the labels Premack assigned to the plastic chips. For example, a typical sign in most signing systems for *woman* is to stroke the cheek slightly below the ear as though tying a bonnet (Roane, 1983). Since bonnets are rarely worn, this sign must be learned just as any spoken word must be learned. In Amer-Ind, the gesture for *woman* is using both hands to make an hour-glass figure, which is immediately understood by almost everyone who sees it (Roane, 1983).

Kirschner, Algozzine, and Abbott (1979) found that Amer-Ind gestures were more intelligible to untrained viewers, were more intelligible after training, and were more intelligible in a two-week follow-up than ASL signs for the same concepts. They conducted this research with university students who were representative of individuals who might at sometime be teaching some form of manual communication to communicatively impaired students. Until recently, most individuals did not know any signing systems unless they were deaf or hard of hearing, had deaf or hard-of-hearing individuals in their households, or worked with deaf or hard-of-hearing individuals. Mayberry (1976) pointed out that certain signing systems might be easier for students to learn and for instructors to teach. The following is a modification of a manual communication system hierarchy suggested by Kirschner et al. (1979), which is ordered from highly structured to nonlinguistic communicative gestures:

I. Spoken language
II. Ameslan and/or variations
  A. Linguistics of Visual English (LOVE)
  B. Signing Exact English (SEE 2)
  C. Seeing Essential English (SEE 1)
  D. Finger spelling
  E. Signed English (Siglish)
  F. American Sign Language (Ameslan)
III. American Indian Sign (Amer-Ind)
IV. Undifferentiated pointing and signing

COMBINED COMMUNICATION SYSTEMS

While it is possible to rely on a single mode of communication (e.g., writing), in actual practice that is rarely ever the case. Normally, when a person speaks, much of what is communicated is communicated visually, as well as auditorily. This is accomplished via facial expressions, gestures, and other forms of body language. Multimodal or multisensory instructional programs have been used with considerable success with moderately to severely handicapped individuals for over 40 years (Fernald, 1943). The term *total communication* has been used more recently to differentiate between specific communication training programs as opposed to referring to overall instructional programs. Normally, total communication involves the visual, auditory, and motor modalities in order to facilitate language acquisition in nonspeaking individuals (Woolman, 1980). This has certainly been true of signing and speaking simultaneously while communicating with deaf individuals.

Kent (1974) and Schaeffer, Musil, and Kollinzas (1980) have developed fine programs for moderately to severely communicatively impaired nonspeaking students, using a total communication approach. Bricker and Bricker (1974) combined objects with gestures that depicted the functions of the objects in order to facilitate the receptive language of severely retarded children. Clark, Moores, and Woodcock (1975a, 1975b) combined speaking, signing, and rebuses in the *Minnesota Early Language Development Sequence*. The meaning was demonstrated by presenting real objects and pictures.

Communication boards are also examples of multimodal communication systems (Moores, 1980). In addition to the words presented in Table 7-1, communication boards may combine letters, numbers, words, rebuses, Bliss symbols, or abstract shapes similar to those used by the Premacks. Computer technology provides the means of adding moving graphics and sound with communication boards. Computers are excellent vehicles for combined communication modes. These will be discussed in Chapter 8.

ADVANTAGES AND DISADVANTAGES OF ALTERNATIVE COMMUNICATION FORMS

ADVANTAGES. The main advantage of an alternative communication form is obvious: a previously noncommunicative individual often learns to communicate. Auditory-vocal individuals are usually unaware of how much of their communication is actually visual-motor. Gestures, facial expressions, and general body language are used to complement the spoken words. These natural gestures are semantically based, as are Bliss symbols and Amer-Ind. Thus, they are readily understood within any given context.

However, many of the visual-motor systems are as abstract as most spoken and written words and, thus, require a comparable level of perceptual and cognitive abilities. Nevertheless, they are useful techniques for many moderately to severely communicatively impaired individuals, particularly those who have auditory processing deficits but are visually strong. Furthermore, there are instances in which visual communication can be thought of as prompts which are used to establish vocal verablization and gradually faded out completely.

Another advantage of many of the visual modes is the constancy of the message. A written word, a plastic chip, or a Bliss symbol can remain constant until the viewer gets the message. This is not true of the spoken word which is literally gone a fraction of a second after it is uttered. The same applies to visual-motor communication forms such as fingerspelling, manual signing, or gesturing. The thing to consider is the possibility that many communicatively impaired individuals may process and produce communication better on a spatial rather than a temporal dimension.

Furthermore, as mentioned on the section on physical prompting in Chapter 3, it is extremely difficult to physically prompt speaking, but it is fairly simple to physically prompt alternative forms of communication.

DISADVANTAGES. Just as the main advantage of alternative communication forms is obvious, so is the main disadvantage: Up to this point in time, they have never received total acceptance. Humans are notoriously unforgiving toward other humans who do not communicate "normally." As parents of communicatively impaired individuals or as professionals or paraprofessionals who work with communicatively impaired individuals, we must recognize that fact and continue working toward educating the nonhandicapped population about how much more normal than handicapped the population labeled "handicapped" is.

Another serious disadvantage is that most of the nonhandicapped population cannot understand or use the alternative communication form. I recall a special education teacher who was teaching her nonspeaking autistic student to sign "apple." An onlooking student said skeptically, "Well, the storeman's not gonna know that means apple." A third disadvantage with some alternative communication forms is the amount of time they take, particularly when attempting to express somewhat complicated ideas.

The fourth difficulty lies in the fact that many of the alternative communication modes require physical, perceptual, cognitive, or symbolization levels that are beyond those experienced by many of the severely communicatively impaired. Alternative forms that are structurally or linguistically based may be as difficult (if not more difficult) to process and produce as speech, depending upon the source of the communicative impairment. Furthermore, some of the alternative communication forms require paraphernalia that is cumbersome and awkward to carry around. Thus, it is rarely used outside of educational or clinical settings.

The final disadvantage is that none of the alternative communication forms can be as flexible, varied, and semantically complete as the spoken language. Nevertheless, since functional communication is the overall objective of CLIP, instructors have a responsibility to utilize whatever strengths each student possesses to make communication a reality for each of their communicatively impaired students.

CHAPTER 8

COMPUTER TECHNOLOGY

JANE Y. MURDOCK

ONE cannot pick up a magazine or a newspaper without being confronted with the fact that the cybernetic age is upon us. The impact of this technology on educating communicatively impaired and other handicapped individuals is undeniable. Over 11 years ago Colby (1973) established a rationale for computer-based treatment for nonspeaking autistic children. His equipment consisted of a television screen and a typewriter-like keyboard. Pressing the keys caused symbols to appear on the screen. The children could actively control the communication by selecting the keys they would press to produce the pictures they wanted to see on the screen. Colby felt that much of the success he and his colleagues had may have been related to the fascination that many autistic individuals have with machines. Furthermore, "The merits of the machine are that it is untiring, predictable, always saying the same thing the same way, never angry, never bored, and controllable — properties which are notoriously lacking in humans." (Colby, 1973, p. 255).

Hannaford and Taber (1982) also pointed to the nonthreatening interaction between the machine and the student as being especially beneficial to handicapped individuals or those who find it difficult to communicate, since they typically experience excessive failure when interacting with people.

It is almost impossible to look over the program of any conference in any area of special education without finding individual presentations or entire programs devoted to research and applications of computer technology. Since 1983 the Council for Exceptional Children, a national organization for special educators and other professionals interested in handicapped and/or gifted children and adults, has held two national topical conferences on technology in special education.

Special thanks to Wilma S. Longstreet for her suggestions and contributions to this chapter.

It is of some concern that a pervasive theme throughout all of these is that the technology is advancing at a much more rapid rate than educators' ability to apply it. It is of further concern that many adults, including teachers, psychologists, and speech pathologists, do not look upon a computer as something that is "nonthreatening." Fortunately, the federal government and the Council for Exceptional Children have recognized the need for special educators and related professionals to become computer literate. Funding through the Department of Education for developing systems, training, and technical assistance related to computer technology has increased dramatically since 1981 (Schiffman, Tobin, & Cassidy-Bronson, 1982).

The Council for Exceptional Children and its Teacher Division are developing a *Training Manual of Microcomputers in Special Education* (Draft) (Kamp, 1983), the draft of which is currently being field-tested. The purpose of the training manual and materials is to train special educators to use microcomputers constructively. Furthermore, many colleges of education and departments of special education and speech pathology and audiology are offering, and in many cases requiring, courses in computer technology for their students. It is particularly pleasing to see the numbers of teachers and other professionals who are flocking to register for these courses at my own university, since the possible applications of these amazing machines are only as diverse as the creativity and technical expertise of those who use them. There is no question that microcomputers could become an integral part of special education in this country. The Council for Exceptional Children is actively involved in promoting the technology and in training special educators and other professionals to use that technology for the benefit of handicapped and gifted students. An entire issue of *Exceptional Children* was devoted to "Microcomputers' Place in Special Education" in October of 1982. The Council for Exceptional Children published Florence M. Taber's book on *Microcomputers in Special Education* in 1983. The entire 1984 Summer issue of *Teaching Exceptional Children* was devoted to "Technology in Special Education." All of these are highly recommended to readers who want more in-depth information than can be presented in a text restricted to moderately to severely communicatively impaired populations.

According to Hannaford and Sloane (1981, p. 48), when a microcomputer is properly programmed, it can do the following for all students:

1. Provide a multisensory approach to learning.
2. Be used to teach a wide range of subject matter.
3. Be used with diverse student populations.
4. Provide direct individualized interactive instruction.
5. Allow a student to learn at his or her own rate.
6. "Remember" student responses.
7. Provide instant feedback.
8. Give a variety of reinforcements.

9. Provide remediation, development, or enrichment depending on the needs of the learner.
10. Provide repetition, drill, and practice in a meaningful manner.
11. Provide diagnostic and prescriptive information to the teachers.
12. Be used as an ideal management and retrieval system for student records, assessment scores, student objectives, and IEP's.
13. Free the teacher from hours of repetitious paper and pencil activities.
14. Provide continuous encouragement to a student and facilitate active participation in the learning process.

Special education and rehabilitation programs are major areas likely to use the computer. According to Cain (1984b), these applications fall into several major, interrelated categories, including communication, problem solving, recreation, and prosthetic devices. Computers can also be used to manage instruction, assist in instruction, and promote creative teaching.

COMMUNICATION

An essential element of a computer technology program for all students is a concept of the computer as a communication tool and as a linguistic device. Computer linguistics refers to how a person "talks" to a computer and how she "receives" information from a computer. In other words, computer linguistics, like auditory-vocal language, includes both receptive and expressive elements (Cain, 1984a).

Expressive Computer Linguistics

A computer is a device that can perform memory and selection functions for the user. It also performs the actual transmission of information, allowing the content of the message to be separated from the actual process of communication. You can communicate with a computer through a variety of data entry and control devices, for example, keyboards and screens, touch screens, telephones, voice-activated systems, voice interactive systems, and hand-controlled devices. A computer also provides the ability to talk with other people through word processing programs, interactive telephone line systems, and interactive cable television systems (Cain, 1984a).

Specifically considering expressive communication of moderately to severely communicatively impaired students, much has been accomplished through the application of computer technology to Bliss symbols (Vanderheiden, 1982; Wertz, Wertz, & Kehrberg, 1983). A significant improvement for Bliss users occurred when Eulenberg and Rahimi combined microprocessor and speech synthesis technology that permitted the user to communicate by producing synthesized English sound from Bliss symbols

(Bennett, 1982). MINSPEAK is another information storage and retrieval system based on concepts and symbols rather than words or letters. According to the Summer 1983 issue of *Current Expressions* (Prentke Romich Company), although MINSPEAK has less than 60 symbols, a sentence of several words can be represented by a sequence of only four of them. For example, if a person presses illustrations of an eye (with a cursive "I," and upper case "I" and a lower case "i" over it), a rope tied in a knot, a telephone, and a person in a wheelchair, a computer would say, "I can't talk and control my wheelchair at the same time." See Appendix B for other examples of portable, computer-based speech synthesizers.

Receptive Aspects of Computer Linguistics

In one sense, the computer may be considered a passive communication device in that it makes no social value judgment regarding the message sender. According to Cain (1984b), some of the most dramatic uses of computer technology for handicapped individuals have occurred when the computer is viewed as an electronic communication system. Students are able to receive information through their strongest modality and they can control the rate of the input. Thus, they can attend to the content of the message rather than to the process of reception. Graphics, sound, and/or voice can be used to enhance comprehension and increase motivation.

PROBLEM-SOLVING COMPETENCY

The ability to function independently or semi-independently in a technological society is directly related to the ability to use that technology to solve problems (Cain, 184a). Thus, it is important to develop the ability of communicatively impaired individuals to use the computer as a problem-solving device. The computer is merely an electronic servant with which a student can have a personal interaction which he controls.

Computer technology systems which have proved effective in teaching problem-solving skills include computer simulations, interactive video systems and LOGO. Computer simulation software and interactive video systems permit practicing learned concepts in situations nearer to the real world than can be experienced in the artificial world of school and textbook (Cain, 1984a). In addition, the medium is interactive and allows for continuous feedback and self-monitoring. Computers also make it easy to keep data current.

LOGO is a recursive computer language most closely related to artifical intelligence computer languages such as LISP. It was developed at the Michigan Institute of Technology primarily for children just learning to use computers. It is heavily dependent on graphics and is a superb way to learn geometry, as well as recursive computer programming.

LOGO turns the microcomputer into an electronic discovery learning system which permits those who have difficulty with oral and written language and with fine motor control an opportunity to learn, think, and try things in individual ways. There is no element of "right" or "wrong" in LOGO. Students are free to explore, create, and self-correct. Errors become the basis of further learning, since the computer never evaluates, but it provides immediate feedback. LOGO fosters analytical reasoning and logical selecting (Cain, 1984a, 1984b; Miller, 1984).

PROSTHETIC DEVICES

The computer may be conceptualized as a prosthetic device that can cause certain symptoms of handicapped individuals to no longer be disabling. The memory and selecting capabilities of the computer make it possible to develop students' ability to use the dynamic qualities of the computer to compensate for neurological, motor, and/or intellectual limitations (Cain, 1984a, 1984b).

Computer applications to educating the physically handicapped population are truly amazing. One needs only to become aware of the literature. Nave, Browning, and Carter (1983) have published *Computer Technology for the Handicapped in Special Education and Rehabilitation: A Resource Guide,* which contains 191 annotated citations from the literature on computers and the handicapped. Vanderheiden (1978) has catalogued over 100 communication devices to aid communicatively impaired and nonspeaking individuals. Vanderheiden and Grilley (1976) categorized communicative devices according to the specific handicap and the consequent selection techniques available.

One of the most exciting and intriguing uses of computer technology is related to improving the communication skills of handicapped individuals through the use of computer-aided prosthetic devices. Remarkable advances have been made with augmentative communication aids for nonspeaking individuals, including those with severe cerebral palsy or other motor impairments. The output mode(s) can be visual, verbal, or both. The selection methods vary according to the ability of the communicatively impaired student. Some students are capable of using a standard keyboard. Others need expanded keyboards which can utilize such devices as mouth or head-mounted light pens to select letters or other symbols. There are also foot, head, chin, or brow switches, joysticks, and sip-and-puff straws that make selections by stopping a cursor (i.e., a small blinking light) as it moves across a matrix display to the desired character (Luttner, 1981; Vanderheiden, 1981). These aids have advanced to the point of a Panasonic hand-held portable communication device that allows the user to quickly and easily display messages (Damasco & Foulds, 1982).

Computer-generated speech can be prerecorded or synthesized speech. Since prerecorded speech is prespoken, it has a limited vocabulary. The sound, however, is natural and easy to perceive, and cassette tapes can be turned on by the microcomputer at the appropriate times. These serve well and are very inexpensive. Synthesized speech is considerably more expensive than prerecorded cassette tapes. An advantage to synthesized speech, however, is that it is not pre-established, therefore, the vocabulary is unlimited and may be utilized as needed rather than sequentially as would be required if the less expensive tape recorder were utilized. However, synthesized sound is robotic and difficult to understand. Appendix B provides a list of some of the companies that produce commercially available communication devices (Bristow, 1983).

According to Spring (1984), speech recognition by a computer is, as of this writing, far from being perfect. The computer has to "learn" the vocal and speech patterns of the speaker. For a very limited set of commands, the computer can be set up to recognize most voice commands, but if a broad range of commands is to be utilized by several voices, then there is still a great deal of development needed. My own experience with this has been very limited, but I found that slight variations in pronunciation resulted in failure on the part of the computer to interpret responses correctly. Obviously, this will vary considerably with the quality of available equipment.

A human can understand most others who speak the same language and can also understand computers. A computer must be trained to the intonation, enunciation, and inflection patterns of each speaker in order to understand. This is an extremely limiting factor for those communicatively impaired individuals who cannot read or recognize visual symbols in order to interact with the computer. Furthermore, there are many communicatively impaired individuals who have extremely erratic vocal patterns, for example, those with athetoid cerebral palsy. Voice recognition will be one of the most fantastic breakthroughs in computer technology. Imagine the programming possibilities for students who cannot read or recognize letters when a computer can "listen" and provide the same feedback and reinforcement it can presently provide for visual-motor input. According to Trachtman (1984), this may not be too far in the future in view of the fact that talking word processors have already been developed by Laura Meyers and Teresa Rosegrant, two linguists and early childhood educators who are dedicated to making communication possible for severely communicatively impaired children.

RECREATIONAL TOOL

Computer technology makes it possible to simulate recreational alternatives. The computer is the only truly "interactive" recreational electronic media. It is very worthwhile to develop handicapped students' ability to use the computer and computer gaming devices as leisure time activities. They can be used individually or in group situations. They can be used simply as games or as instructional games. They can simulate sports that many handicapped students could not participate in otherwise. Computer-linked video systems are ideal for providing multisensory recreational activities. Furthermore, there is a lagniappe effect associated with computer games. Since many nonhandicapped students spend much of their leisure time (and money) playing video games, it is important to the normalization process for handicapped students to learn how to participate in these activities also (Cain, 1984a, 1984b).

USING A MICROCOMPUTER TO MANAGE INSTRUCTION

There are many burdensome and time-consuming clerical chores for special educators, speech pathologists, psychologists, and others who work with handicapped students. Many of these are the result of the legal mandates of Public Law 94-142 which require: (1) an individualized education plan (IEP) for every handicapped student, (2) tracking students from the time of their initial referral until they are appropriately placed and making certain that appropriate placement occurs within specified timelines set forth in state and federal regulations, and (3) grouping students on the basis of individual needs identified in their IEP's.

Without having any prior computer experience, you can make excellent use of a microcomputer to plan and manage communication and language instruction by purchasing and using appropriate software. Some of the sources for software are included in Appendix C. For those of you who are more sophisticated, develop your own programs using Basic or, in some cases, word processing programs. In my experience, the latter are considerably less flexible than other programs, but they do provide adequate data storage and graphing capabilities. (All of the graphs in Chapter 4 were initiated through a word processing program and printed on a Diablo printer.)

Package programs such as electronic spread sheets and data-based filing systems might be effectively used, depending on the system of records being developed for the handicapped student. Lotus 123 is an electronic spread sheet that allows both quantitative and cursive data to be categorized and stored. Graphs also can be developed based on the stored quantitative data.

Several programs have been developed to assist with individual education programs. For example, Brown (1982) discusses Computer-Assisted Management of Educational Objectives (CAMEO), which she reports can minimize preparatory work on IEP's and reduce clerical time enormously, without compromising the ability to address individual student needs. Project RECIPE (Research Exchange for Computerized Individualized Programs of Education) is a nationally validated instructional management system designed to help teachers and other professionals create and implement individualized education programs (Bailey & Raimondi, 1984; Bell & Cady, 1984). A computer-managed project developed in Maryland to print IEP's, track individual due process requirements, and create instructional groups has been selected as a national training model and exchange program through the Council of Administrators of Special Education (CASE) (Cassidy-Bronson, Miller, & Slaughter, 1984). AIMSTAR (Hasselbring & Hamlett, 1984) is another computer program designed to store and graph student data and assist teachers in evaluating programs.

COMPUTER-ASSISTED INSTRUCTION

For the uninitiated, computer-assisted instruction (CAI) seems to be synonymous with computer technology. However, it is obvious from the foregoing that computer technology can assist handicapped students in many other ways, in addition to direct, interactive instruction when the student is on-line with a computer. The microcomputer is a great improvement over the mainframe computers that were hooked into classrooms in the 1960's, both in terms of cost and utilization. The micro is also a vast improvement in terms of the interactive environment that it provides. Mainframes were primarily batch oriented, with little interaction between user and computer. Furthermore, educators can use the available CAI software quite readily which was not the case with mainframe computers (Budoff & Hutten, 1982).

Computer-assisted instruction that is appropriate for moderately to severely communicatively impaired students can be: (1) drill and practice, (2) tutorial, (3) educational games, (4) simulation, and (5) problem solving. Drill and practice is the most common and is designed to integrate, reinforce, and otherwise supplement previously learned material. Tutorial programs present material in a programmed format. The student moves at his own pace, advancing as he masters the material and otherwise branching to review or remedial segments. Educational games are designed to motivate students and develop general problem-solving strategies. Simulations attempt to bridge the gap between the real world and contrived learning environments. As mentioned earlier, computer simulations and interactive video systems can be used effectively to teach problem-solving skills. LOGO may also be used as a problem-solving program for communicatively impaired and other handicapped students.

CAI Software

In addition to the lag between advances in computer technology and technical expertise on the part of educators and other professionals, which was mentioned ealier, there is another serious problem related specifically to computer-assisted instruction: The software, which is the very heart of a computer-assisted learning system, is generally poor. According to Schiffman et al. (1982, p. 425), "Unfortunately, most of the available software is uninspired and little more than a duplication of textbooks and 'print' material." According to Hofmeister (1982, p. 116), "In general, the quality of presently available educational software is very disappointing." According to Hannaford (1983, p. 15), "The greatest difficulty facing the use of microcomputers in special education, however, lies not with the resistance and caution of educators, it lies with the software or courseware." In addition to these general problems, there is a dire shortage of software developed for moderately to severely communicatively impaired individuals. You will have a great deal more flexibility if you can do some programming yourself.

Easy-to-Develop Software

You can develop your own software, individualized to your own students. You do not have to spend years studying computer technology or computer languages to do this. This following is a simplified overview of how you might write a program using the most elementary knowledge of Basic with a TRS-80 (Models I, III, or IV) microcomputer. I have selected Basic as the language because, as far as I can determine, it is used for educationl programs more than any other computer language. I have selected a TRS-80 microcomputer because that is the kind I have. (However, the program does work on other computers, such as the IBM-PC and the Zenith-100. I think that it might also work on some models of the Apple if the CLS command were changed to HOME.) This program is written for readers who know absolutely nothing about microcomputers or programming. You can play with this program, modify it, and make it work, even if you're one of those who is scared to touch the micro's in the airport lobbies.

HOW TO BEGIN. Turn the machine on. The switch on the TRS-80 is underneath on the right-hand side near the front. However, switch placement can vary, and that may not be the location for the model you're using months or years after this writing. Often, they're located on the right at the back. Don't let a machine make you feel foolish! If you can't find the switch to turn it on, ask for help. After the machine is switched on, a red light will appear and you may also hear a whirring sound, depending on whether your microcomputer is equipped with a disk drive. NEVER INSERT OR REMOVE A DISKETTE WHILE A RED LIGHT IS ON!

When the light goes off, insert a diskette that has been initialized for Basic programming on a TRS-80 in drive 0 (the bottom drive) and close the door securely. This diskette is referred to as "TRSDOS." If you do not have an initialized diskette, go to the nearest Radio Shack and they will help you. Actually, you do not need TRSDOS to work in Basic on the TRS-80, Model III, since

Basic has been placed in ROM as part of the hardward configuration of the micro. However, disk Basic is more powerful than simple Basic. Now the machine is on, the diskette is inserted in drive 0, and the door over the drive is securely closed. Press the orange, inset button on the upper right-hand side of the keyboard. This is the reset button. The red light will occur again. A message will appear on the screen with copyright information and the direction "ENTER DATE (MM/DD/YY)?" Enter the date in that format: 05/30/84. Press the ENTER key on the right side of the keyboard.

The screen will ask for the time, but simply press ENTER again. The message "TRSDOS Ready" will appear on the screen. Type "Basic" and press ENTER. The screen will now ask a series of questions (How many files? Memory size?). Simply press ENTER as each question appears until you get the message "READY" and a ">" on the left-hand side of the screen. The microcomputer is now ready for you to begin entering your program.

LINE NUMBERS. Following the ">," type a number to begin each line of information you want to put into your program. It is wise to use line numbers in increments of at least 10 so that lines can be inserted to modify the program. As you begin entering your program, don't number lines more closely. There is no benefit to close numbering and doing so makes later modification more difficult. The following program began with all lines in increments of 10. I typed the lines into this chapter exactly as they appear on the final version of the program to give you an indication of the modifications that occurred. Line numbers are very important in Basic because a program moves sequentially through the line numbers unless directed to do otherwise. Furthermore, a program line may be substituted by typing its number followed by the new line. After you finish typing all the information you want on a line, press the ENTER key in order to have the microcomputer perform the commands you have put in.

CLS STATEMENT. Typing "CLS" will clear or erase the screen. This statement makes it possible to limit the number of lines on the screen or printed page and allows the message to appear from the top to the bottom of the screen without scrolling. The CLEAR key on the keyboard can immediately accomplish the same thing, but it cannot be a part of a program. You can start a program by typing "CLS" on the first line:

```
10 CLS
15 C=0
16 N=0
18 D=0
```

Observe that lines 15, 16, and 18 were inserted. The reason for this will be explained later.

REMARK STATEMENTS. At the beginning of your program you can put in any information you think you might need to identify the program or remind you of things you might wish to know about the program by typing "REM" followed by whatever you wish. For example:

```
20 REM /z/ PLURALS – BODY PARTS
```

PRINT STATEMENTS. Typing "PRINT" can cause your computer to act like a calculator or, when followed by quotation marks around words, to act like a typewriter. For the purposes of this program it will be used to cause the computer to act like a typewriter. Now to insert the next line:

```
30 PRINT "HELLO. MY NAME IS MICRO. BUT YOU CAN CALL
   ME MIKE."
40 PRINT "WHAT IS YOUR NAME?"
```

INPUT STATEMENTS. These usually follow questions. They allow the student and the computer to interact with each other. After asking the student's name, provide an INPUT statement:

```
50 INPUT N$
60 PRINT " NICE MEETING YOU, ";N$;"."
65 PRINT
70 PRINT "I CAN HELP YOU TALK TO PEOPLE."
75 PRINT
80 PRINT " WOULD YOU LIKE THAT?"
```

"N$" allows the computer to accept a word or a string of words for the input. A letter without the "$" allows the computer to accept number(s). When PRINT is not followed by any text, as in lines 65 and 75 which were inserted after viewing the program, PRINT acts as though it were a command to skip a line. The logic is simple: The computer is told to "PRINT" but has no information about what to print, so it automatically saves a space between the text that was specified in the preceding and following lines.

Notice the spacing and punctuation in the commands given in lines 60 through 80. There are quotation marks around everything that will appear on the screen when the student is running the program. Any punctuation inside of those quotation marks will be printed. Thus, line 60 has a comma before the first close quotation mark appears. There is a space between this comma and the quotation mark in order to preserve that space in the printed text. Semicolons surround the "N$" which, if you recall, was the INPUT statement following a request for the student's name. The semicolons will not appear on the screen but are used to indicate that what does appear on the screen goes into the next available space. A period is placed between quotation marks in order for this sentence to be punctuated correctly. Additional spacing, such as that between the first quotation mark and the beginning of the greeting, simply centers the message on the screen better. (The remainder of the program as it is printed in this chapter will not attempt to accommodate the spacing of the original program because publication guidelines recommend 55 spaces per line

line for this text and the screen on the TRS-80 Model III microcomputer has 64 spaces.) With the foregoing punctuation and spacing considerations, if the student typed in "SAM" for the INPUT N$ statement, the computer would type out:

NICE MEETING YOU, SAM.

I CAN HELP YOU TALK.

WOULD YOU LIKE THAT?

Since there is another question, there usually follows another INPUT statement.

```
90 INPUT A$
95 C=C+1
```

"C=C+1" causes the computer to count each answer that is input in response to the question in line 80. Line 15 was inserted at the beginning of the program to ensure that "C" will start at zero. This must be at the beginning of the program so that no routine will return to it and interfere with the following counting sequence:

$$C=0 \rightarrow C+1=1 \rightarrow C+1=2 \rightarrow C+1=3$$

As you can see, the quantity of C is increased by adding 1 each time the sequence is repeated.

IF-THEN STATEMENTS. These always go together. They allow the computer to respond in certain ways according to the student's input. For example:

```
100 IF A$="no" THEN 630
105 IF A$="NO" THEN 630
```

This statement will move the program from line 90 to line 630 if the student's input was "NO" or "no" in either upper or lower case type. Follow lines 630 through 670 to see how the computer prints regrets on the screen, directs the student to seek assistance from his teacher, and ends the program. (I apologize to the reader because line 630 is several pages forward in this text. After much deliberation, I determined that this inconvenience was warranted in order to have the narrative explanation adjacent to each new statement as it appeared in the program.)

```
110 IF A$="yes" THEN 170
115 IF A$="YES" THEN 170
```

This statement will move the program from line 90 to line 170 if the student's input was "YES" or "yes" in either upper or lower case type. In response to line 170, the computer expresses pleasure and then moves sequentially through line 280 with the program's instructions, question, and multiple-choice alternatives. Since there is no guarantee that the answer will be "yes" or "no," you will need more PRINT statements, but first you need another IF-THEN statement.

```
120 IF C>3 THEN 640
130 PRINT: PRINT "I CAN'T UNDERSTAND YOUR ANSWER.":
    PRINT: PRINT "PLEASE ANSWER 'YES' OR 'NO.'": FOR
    TL=1 TO 1000: NEXT TL
135 IF C=1 THEN 70
140 PRINT: PRINT "WOULD YOU LIKE ME TO HELP YOU
    TALK?": PRINT
145 IF C=2 THEN 70
150 PRINT "PLEASE ANSWER 'YES' OR 'NO.'"
160 IF C=3 THEN 70
```

The IF-THEN statement in line 120 tells the computer to go to line 640 if the student has failed to respond with a "yes" or "no" in three trials. After the message in the PRINT statement in line 640 appears on the screen, the student is directed to seek assistance from her teacher and the program ends. Lines 135, 145, and 160 return the program to line 70, providing the three opportunities for the student to accept or reject interacting with the computer. Lines 130, 140, and 150 repeat the question and response instructions.

By using the colon between instructions, line 130 combines statements that will be utilized sequentially. The reason for such combinations is to save memory space for programming rather than taking it up with line numbers. Before combining statements on a line, consider carefully whether any statement in the combination will be needed independently later on in the program. If the answer is "yes," then put that statement on a line with its own number, because designating the line number is the only way you can tell the computer how to find it. Otherwise, you can put up to 255 characters on a single line as long as you separate each statement with a colon.

FOR-NEXT STATEMENTS. Line 130 also contains a FOR-NEXT statement that requires some explanation. These statements are useful when you want to repeat a procedure several times. Also, they are used to cause the computer to count or do other things you request. The FOR-NEXT statement in line 130 is a time loop that causes the computer to slow down, allowing the student time to read the screen and make decisions. The computer is literally counting in place, going nowhere. The higher the number is, the more time the student will have. This is a particularly useful function for moderately to severely communicatively impaired students, but it is one that must be adjusted carefully to meet individual requirements. There may be a near optimum presentation rate for each individual that depends upon: (1) how long it takes to process information, (2) how good the short-term memory is, and (3) how well a person attends

(Murdock & Sabrio, 1983). When you play around with this program, be sure to vary the time loops so that you can get a feeling for what can be done with them to accommodate each of your own students. You can do this by editing the line or by typing the line number again with a greater or lesser time loop (e.g., FOR TL=1 TO 50 or FOR TL=1 TO 2500, etc.).

Now, on with the program, assuming that a student responded with a "yes" within three opportunities and the program was directed to line 170.

```
170 PRINT "WONDERFUL! THAT MAKES ME VERY HAPPY.":
    FOR TL=1 TO 2000: NEXT TL: CLS
180 PRINT "I'LL KEEP TALKING TO YOU BY WRITING"
190 PRINT "ON THIS SCREEN. YOU ANSWER ME BY"
200 PRINT "PRESSING THE LETTER ON MY KEYBOARD"
210 PRINT "THAT MATCHES THE RIGHT ANSWER."
220 PRINT "LET'S TRY IT.": FOR TL=1 TO 2500: NEXT TL
230 IF N=> 3 THEN 650 ELSE CLS
240 PRINT "WHEN WE TALK ABOUT ONE HAND, WE SAY"
245 PRINT
250 PRINT "'HAND.' WHAT DO WE SAY WHEN WE"
255 PRINT
260 PRINT "TALK ABOUT MORE THAN ONE HAND?"
265 PRINT
270 PRINT "A. HAND", "B. HANDS", "C. HEET", "D. HANDES"
```

The commas outside of the quotation marks in line 270 place each of these four choices equally across the screen. The use of the comma invokes a built-in tabulation. The screen is conceptually divided into four columns. The comma sends the cursor to the next column as opposed to the semicolon which advances it to the next space.

```
275 PRINT
280 PRINT "(CHOOSE A, OR B, OR C, OR D)"
300 INPUT B$
330 IF B$="B" THEN 500
340 IF B$="A" THEN 364
350 IF B$="C" THEN 364
360 IF B$="D" THEN 364
362 GO TO 680
364 N=N+1
```

Lines 330 through 360 direct the program when a student responds to the instructions in line 280. Line 362 directs the program when a student is not following instructions. Line 364 is a counting line so that the student can be prompted appropriately according to the prompting procedures recommended in CLIP. Note the following:

```
366 IF N=1 THEN 370
367 IF N=2 THEN 420
368 IF N=3 THEN 460
370 CLS: PRINT "NOT QUITE."
375 PRINT
380 PRINT "REMEMBER WHAT YOU SAY WHEN YOU TALK"
385 PRINT
390 PRINT "ABOUT MORE THAN ONE EAR?"
395 PRINT
400 PRINT "LET'S TRY AGAIN.": FOR TL=1 TO 2500: NEXT TL:
    GOTO 230
```

GOTO STATEMENTS. A GOTO statement is another way of telling the computer not to carry out the commands in numerical order. IF-THEN and GOTO statements are often used together. The GOTO statement in line 362 directs the program to line 680 in order to repeat the instructions three times if the student fails to follow them. The GOTO statement in line 400 directs the program back to line 230 to determine whether the student has already completed the third trial when responding correctly to the instructions.

```
420 PRINT "NOT QUITE, ";N$;", WHEN WE TALK ABOUT
    MORE THAN ONE EAR,"
425 PRINT
430 PRINT "WE SAY 'EARS."
435 PRINT
440 PRINT "NOW LET'S TRY AGAIN."
445 FOR TL=1 TO 1500: NEXT TL: CLS: GOTO 230
460 CLS: PRINT "SORRY, "N$;", WHEN WE TALK ABOUT
    MORE THAN ONE HAND,"
465 PRINT
470 PRINT "WE SAY 'HANDS.'"
475 FOR TL=1 TO 1500: NEXT TL
477 PRINT
480 PRINT "RAISE YOUR HAND NOW SO THAT YOUR
    TEACHER CAN HELP YOU."
490 GO TO 620
```

Line 490 directs the program to END after the student has failed to respond correctly and has been instructed to seek assistance.

```
500 N=N+1: CLS: PRINT "GREAT! YOU SAID 'HANDS.'"
505 PRINT
510 PRINT "WHEN YOU TALK ABOUT MORE THAN ONE
    HAND, YOU ADD AN 'S'"
515 PRINT
```

```
520 PRINT "HAND→HANDS"
525 PRINT
530 PRINT "RAISE YOUR HAND, ";N$;". TELL YOUR
    TEACHER YOU HAVE"
540 IF N=1 THEN 570
550 IF N=2 THEN 590
560 IF N=3 THEN 610
570 PRINT "JUST EARNED 15 POINTS!"
580 END
590 PRINT "JUST EARNED 10 POINTS!"
600 END
610 PRINT "JUST EARNED 5 POINTS!"
620 END
```

Lines 500 through 620 allow for different reinforcers for a student who took one, two, or three trials to respond correctly.

```
630 PRINT "I'M SORRY, ";N$;". THAT MAKES ME SAD."
635 PRINT
640 PRINT "MAYBE WE CAN TALK LATER."
645 PRINT
650 PRINT "PLEASE RAISE YOUR HAND SO THAT YOUR"
660 PRINT "TEACHER CAN HELP YOU."
670 END
```

Lines 630 through 670 provide the computer's response to the student who answered "NO" (I don't want you to help me talk to people). Lines 640 through 670 provide the computer's response to the student who fails to answer "YES" or "NO" in three trials.

```
680 D=D+1
690 PRINT "THAT IS NOT A CHOICE. REMEMBER YOU MUST
    PRESS 'A' OR 'B' OR 'C' OR 'D'"
700 FOR TL=1 TO 1500: NEXT TL: CLS
710 IF D=3 THEN 650 ELSE 220
```

Lines 680 through 710 provide a means of escape for a student who does not understand the instructions or otherwise fails to respond appropriately within three trials. After the third opportunity to respond by pressing "A," "B," "C," or "D," the student is directed to raise her hand and ask the teacher for assistance. Line 710 directs the program according to how many times the student has failed to follow instructions.

LIST. This is a command that allows you to review your program. Do not type a line number. Simply type LIST immediately after the ">." This will cause the computer to display the entire program, which will scroll through rapidly, only allowing the last 15 or 20 lines to remain on the screen for your perusal. However, you can select the lines you wish to review by typing the specific line or lines (e.g., LIST 10-60).

RUN. Now for the fun (or trials and tests, as the case may be). Typing "RUN" without a line number will cause your program to do just that. If there are problems, many of them will be evident immediately. For example, "Syntax error in line 160" may appear on the screen. Then 160 appears. Simply press the space bar to reveal the line and correct the error. Sometimes the line number does not appear. When this occurs, type "LIST 160" so that you can correct the syntax error. Often, these are simply misspelled words.

However, the computer cannot identify all of the possible problems for you. You want to check your program carefully to see how it will react to things that students might do. For example, in the foregoing program, I initially did not consider the possibility that a student might respond to the first question, "Would you like that?" with something other than a "yes" or "no." When that occurred to me, I changed the program so that it would request the student to answer with a "yes" or "no" response if she failed to do so on the first trial. This sort of thing is one of the great advantages of doing your own programming. You have the ability to get into the program to make it better as flaws are discovered and as your students progress.

The foregoing is a very simple program, which could be written by a novice. That was done for two reasons: (1) I was the only available author, and (2) the input statements would be clear to those of you who are novice readers. The logic in such a simple program is clear. It is obvious from the above that there are great expansion capabilities and versatility using Basic programming. For example, a program normally would not end after one correct response but would continue with several similar but progressively more difficult problems.

One of the more exciting adaptations is that a prerecorded tape recorder can be connected to some microcomputers, including a TRS-80, and the words will be spoken to the student as they are printed on the screen. This makes it usable for nonreaders. Some programs have been so simplified that the student only needs to press the space bar (or any other key) to signal the program to continue. Hopefully, in the not-too-distant future, the computer's receptive language will be perfected to the extent that it can respond reliably to spoken input.

For those whose appetites have been whetted, refer to Appendix C for a resource guide to periodicals, books, organizations, resource groups, networks, projects, and clearinghouses which you can select from and investigate for further information. As I said earlier, "the possible applications of these amazing machines are only as diverse as the creativity and technical expertise of those who use them."

CREATIVE TEACHING AND COMPUTER TECHNOLOGY

Perhaps creativity on the part of communication and language instructors is the necessary ingredient if we are to maximize the potential of computer technology. Trachtman (1984) reported on the work being done by Laura Meyers and Teresa Rosegrant. Meyers, who is a specialist in linguistics and child language development, has had considerable success using computers to help children learn to speak. For example, a 2½-year-old Down's syndrome child was so delighted that he could generate his own words with a speech synthesizer that he said 25 new words in the first session. He had learned only five words in the previous year.

Meyers eventually designed a system called "Programs for Early Acquisition of Language" (PEAL) which, according to Trachtman, has a flat touch-sensitive membrane board with large squares for pictures, symbols, and words. It is connected to an Apple II computer and an Echo II speech synthesizer. Rosegrant and Meyers together have developed talking word processors. They have little or no faith in CAI per se. They think that much of their success is due to their software, which is developed specifically to meet the needs of their clients.

Some of the children can only touch the squares with their feet initially, but Meyers reports that it is not unusual for these children who begin to gain some control over their environments to progress rapidly to hand control and speaking. As she says: "What we can do is immediately give them the ability to talk through the computer. And what happens in many cases is that they start to talk with their mouths. At first they thought, 'I'm a failure, I can't talk.' And all of a sudden they think, 'I can.' And the words just start to come out" (Trachtman, 1982, p. 48).

Appendix A

ORDERED LIST OF ENVIRONMENTALLY USEFUL WORDS

BARBARA V. HARTMANN

THESE word lists were prepared to be helpful in planning remedial speech and language programs. The lists contain words with vowls and consonants in the initial, medial and final position in words. These word lists are generally ordered from easier to more difficult to pronounce. The sounds are approximately ordered from early to later acquisition for most children.

VOWELS in the INITIAL position, simple words (See [h] list also):

[o]
oh
old
open
okay
only
[ẹ]
ape
eight
ate
end
empty
[ae]
ant
ad
apple
[a]
on
arm
air
over
[a]
I
eye
I('m)
ice
[ʌ]
up
under
all
off
[I]
icky
in
inside
Indian
its (me, big, etc.)
itch
[i]
eat
easy
[au]
ow
out
ouch
outside
[ɛ]
egg
[ə]
again
[əi]
oil
[ɪ]
eat
ear

Adapted from: Murdock, J. Y., & Hartmann, B. *A Language Development Program: Imitative Gestures to Basic Syntactic Structures.* Salt Lake City: Word Making Productions, 1975.

CONSONANTS in initial, medial and final-position, simple words:

/n/

INITIAL

no
new
knee
nine
name
nap
nut
net
night
neck
nail
knife
nose
nest
nurse
knitting
needle
number
nickel
napkin
nightgown
newspaper
necklace

MEDIAL

money
penny
pony
honey
peanut
bunny
doughnut
funny
piano
running
raining
Kleenex™

FINAL

in
man
pan
pin
mine
moon
noon
hen
win
ten
can
down
done
gun
fine
fan
sun
run

/m/

INITIAL

my
mine
man
moon
mop
map
meat
make
mad
mud
mess
mouse
mouth
minute
money
mitten
Monday
monkey
moutain
milk
middle
movie
more
motor
mirror
marble
music
mistake
matches
mother

MEDIAL

hammer
mommy
mama
camel
lemon
mailman
milkman
farmer
summer
fireman
tomato
animal
lawn mower

FINAL

arm
name
comb
gum
game
dime
worm
farm
lamb
jam
climb
broom
drum
them
ice cream

/p/

INITIAL

pie
pay
pop

pipe
pot
pan
pen
pin
pig
pull
pill
pail
push
peas
peach
porch
page
purse
pear
park
paste
pants
point
paint
pink
penny
pony
peanut
piano
pickle
pencil
purple
popcorn
puppy
potty
picnic
pocket
pancake
pumpkin
pillow
paper (news)
pepper
parade
parrot
puzzle
package
police
pretty
potato
pajamas
policeman, car

MEDIAL

open
apple
happy
puppy
pumpkin
pepper
paper
diaper
dustpan
jumping
zipper
purple
slipper
computer

FINAL

up
hop
pop
mop
map
top
cup
help
ship
sheep
soap
soup
rope
lamp
grape

/h/

INITIAL

hi
high
hay
how
hoe
who
hop
hen
ham
home
hit
hot
hat
hook
hang
head
hide
hand
help
half
hole
hose
house
hurt
hair (brush)
heart
horse
hammer
happy
hiccup
hot dog
heavy
hello
hurry
hanger
hungry
hundred
hamburger
helicopter

MEDIAL

beehive
downhill
doghouse
dollhouse

rain hat
birdhouse

/t/

INITIAL

tie
toe
two
top
tape
tight
ton
talk
tall
tail
tent
turn
tire
tear
tummy
table
towel
tiger
tickle
ticket
T.V.
toaster
tired
turkey
turtle
Tuesday
teeth (tooth)
twelve
telephone

MEDIAL

eating
mitten
button
tiptoe
kitten
butter
water
doctor
letter
rattle
turtle
lettuce
bathtub
potato
tomato

FINAL

eat
hot
hat
wait
cat
coat
kite
boat
boot
got
ghost
goat
gate
fat
feet
fight
light
sit
want
jet
shirt
salt
robot
peanut
rabbit

/k/

INITIAL

key
cow
cup
cap
come
comb
can
coal
cat
kite
cake
kick
king
call
cold
corn
car
card
cookie
cowboy
cobweb
cupcake
kitten
candy
camel
color
candle
coffee
carrot
camera
keyboard
coffee pot
kitchen
computer

MEDIAL

hockey
hiccough
cocoa
cookie
pocket
bacon
bucket
pumpkin
bookcase
sucker
soccer
package

raincoat
rocket
record
chicken
jacket
broken
napkin

FINAL

neck
make
hook
cook
cake
coke
kick
take
bike
back
book
walk
lake
lock
look
rock
sick
sack
break
block
snake

/f/

INITIAL

foot
fat
feet
fight(ing)
fine
fun(ny)
fan
full
face
fence
four
fork
fast
fix
fly
frog
fridge
five
fifty
fifteen
football
finger
fall down
fish(ing)
fireman
farmer
forty
fourteen
father
feather
flower

MEDIAL

muffin
coffee
waffle
barefoot
waterfall
breakfast
coffeepot
elephant
telephone
grandfather

FINAL

off
half
knife
tough
cough
wolf
laugh
leaf
safe
roof
enough
giraffe

/w/

INITIAL

win
wet
wig
white
wheel
wall
whale
want
walk
wear
warm
worm
work
witch
watch
wagon
walking
window
windy
water
wallet
washing machine
waving
winter
waist
waffle
Wednesday
washcloth
wastebasket
watermelon

MEDIAL

away
awake
towel
sandwich
homework

cobweb
lawn mower

/ŋ/

MEDIAL

hanger
monkey
donkey
finger
hungry
racing car
frying pan
ironing board

FINAL

wing
king
long
sing
ring
wrong
swing
string
eating
painting
washing
fighting
watching
jumping
crying
swimming
sleeping

/b/

INITIAL

bow
bee
bye
boy
bean
bone
bun
boat
boot
beet
bite
book
bike
bank
bang
bag
big
bad
bed
bump
ball
bell
bowl
belt
bus
bush
barn
bear
bird
bench
box
broom
bread
blue
beehive
bottom
button
funny
bucket
butter
bacon
Band-Aid™
bedroom
balloon
bottle
basement
bathroom
birthday
banana
butterfly

MEDIAL

baby
cowboy
elbow
bubble
table
football
rainbow
rabbit
robot
ribbon
teddy bear
keyboard
sandbox
hamburger

FINAL

bib
tub
job
bathrobe
doorknob
cobweb

/g/

INITIAL

go
gum
game
gone
gun
goat
gate
good
goose
gas
give
gift
ghost
girl
guitar
garden
garage

garbage

MEDIAL

buggy
wagon
riger
finger
sugar
hamburger
kangaroo
alligator

FINAL

egg
hug
pig
wig
big
bug
dog
leg
rug
flag
frog
hot dog

/s/

INITIAL

saw
sun
same
soap
soup
sign(ing)
sad
seed
sit
sock
sick
sing
seal
sink
sand
salt
six
sewing
city
soda
sitting
silly
saddle
salad
sofa
seven
sidewalk
summer
cereal
sixteen
scissors
sandwich
seventeen

MEDIAL

icing
messy
pencil
seesaw
bicycle
tricycle
glasses
motorcycle

FINAL

ice
mouse
kiss
bus
gas
face
yes
rice
boots
books
pants
blocks
glass
necklace
suitcase
carrots
purse
horse
nurse
dress
cross

/j/

INITIAL

you
yolk
yawn
young
year
your
yarn
yard
yeast

MEDIAL

yo-yo
onion
canyon
crayon

/d/

INITIAL

do
dumb
dime
duck
dump
down
don't
dog
dig
dad(dy)
dish
doll
door
deer
desk
dance

dirt(y)
dark
diaper
doughnut
donkey
doctor
dinner
dollar
dentist
dessert
downstairs
different

MEDIAL

body
hot dog
window
pudding
candy
candle
under
garden
ladder
ready
radio
soda
saddle
Indian

FINAL

mud
mad
head
hide
bed
good
hand
old
seed
sad
read
red
ride
bird
card

/ ℓ /

INITIAL

lie
low
lamb
lip
lake
light
lock
look
luck(y)
lick
long
loud
lid
leg
lamp
lion
land
leaf
life
laugh
loose
less
large
learn
lost
left
love
lone
lemon
lady
lightening
lettuce
ladder
letter
lizard
lifeguard
library
lawn mower
living room

MEDIAL

pillow
elbow
wallet
toilet
balloon
police
sailor
salad
ruler
Jell-O™
elephant
eleven
telephone
alligator
calendar
valentine
chocolate
watermelon

FINAL

owl
nail
mail
whale
wheel
wall
tail
ball
bell
shell
towel
camel
pencil
shovel
apple
bubble
pickle
candle
rattle
saddle
turtle
whistle

/ɹ/

INITIAL

room
robe
rope
rain(ing)
run
right
rat
root
rug
rag
rock
rake
wrong
ride
road
red
read
roof
rice
race
rose
writing
record
rocket
robot
ready
radio
ruler
rattle
rainbow
raincoat
raisin
return key
refrigerator
rollerskate

MEDIAL

arrow
around
hurry
Mary
merry
parrot
parade
carry
carrot
berry
sorry
cheery
story
jumping rope
giraffe
garage

/ ɜ /

INITIAL

earn
early
earth

MEDIAL

worm
hurt
dirt
work
burn
bird
girl
shirt
purse
nurse
first
church
third
shirt
curtain
turkey
turtle
purple
circle
circus
cursor
iron
thirty
Thursday
syrup

/ ə /

POSTVOCALIC

arm
more
car
hair
here
near
warm
horn
pear
bear
where
tire
car
deer
door
fire
four
jar
chair
store
heart
park
barn
corn
card
yarn
dark
farm
fork
short
horse
army
party
guitar
garden
marble
airplane

FINAL

under

hammer
motor
paper
pepper
water
tiger
bigger
butter
dinner
hanger
diaper
doctor
farmer
number
finger
letter
ladder
color
dollar
summer
ruler
shower
zipper
sister
scissors
picture
teacher
mother
father
feather
flower
spider
sweater
cracker
brother
peanut butter
December
computer

/ʃ/

INITIAL

show
shoe
sheep
ship
shut
sheet
shoot
shout
shell
share
shirt
short(s)
shopping
shower
shadow
shampoo
sugar
shovel
shoulder

MEDIAL

ashes
ocean
machine
cushion
tee shirt
washing
dishes
fishing
sunshine

FINAL

push
wash
dish
fish
brush
toothbrush

/τʃ/

INITIAL

chew
chop
chain
chin
chalk
cheek
chair
cheese
church
check(ers)
chimney
chicken
chilly
child(ren)
chest
cherry
chocolate

MEDIAL

ketchup
kitchen
pitcher
teacher
potato chip
rocking chair

FINAL

match
peach
watch
witch
catch
bench
lunch
church
sandwich
hopscotch
spinach
french fries

/δʒ/

INITIAL

jaw
jam
gym
jeep
June
jet
joke
jump(ing, rope)
juice

junk
jeans
jacks
jelly
Jell-O
July
giant
jungle
giraffe

MEDIAL

engine (fire)
magic
angel
p. j.'s
soldier
orange juice
pajamas
garbage can
vegetable
refrigerator
jungle gym

FINAL

hedge
badge
page
cage
fudge
bridge
judge
orange
cabbage
garbage

/v/

INITIAL

van
vet
vase
voice
veil
vest
very
violin
valentine
vitamin
V.W.
vacation
volcano
vegetable

MEDIAL

oven
movie
waving
T.V.
shovel
over
Levi's™
seven
beaver
gravy
elevator
overalls
envelope
seventeen
television

FINAL

hive (beehive)
move
give
love
five
stove
glove (boxing)
twelve

/z/

INITIAL

zoo
zip
zero
zipper
zebra

MEDIAL

easy
busy
music
lazy
lizzard
razor
freezer
clothes
scissors
magazine

FINAL

eyes
hose
beans
rose
bears
birds
cheese
skills
please
gloves
flags
frogs
lemons
mittens
kittens
cookies
onions
bubbles
scissors
matches
cherries
crackers
crayons
french fries
bananas
pajamas

/θ/

INITIAL

thumb
thin
thick
thank(s) (you)
thorn

third
throw
through (threw)
three
thread
throat
thimble
thirty
thermos
thousand
Thursday
thanksgiving

MEDIAL

bathtub
toothpick
something
toothpaste
bathrobe
toothbrush
twenty-three

FINAL

mouth
month
with
tooth
teeth
south
smooth

/ ð /

INITIAL

the
they
them
then
that
this
their (there)
these
those
themselves

MEDIAL

other
mother
weather
father
feather
leather
brother
rhythm
smoother
another
together
bathing suit
grandmother
grandfather
stepmother
stepfather

FINAL

bathe (s, ed)
wreathe
breathe
smooth

/ ℓ / *Blends*

/bl/

blue
block
blind

/pl/

play
plane
plate

/gl/

glue
glad
glass
glasses

/kl/

climb
clap
clock
clothes

/fl/

fly
float
flag
floor
flower

/s/ *Blends*

/sn/

snow
snake
sniff
snail
sneeze

/sk/

sky
ski
skip
skate
skunk
school
scouts
skirt

/sp/

spoon
spot
spill
space
spider

/st/

stay
stop
step
steak
stuck
stick(y)
stamp
stove
star
store
story
stocking

/sm/

smoke
small
smile
smart
smooth

/sw/

swim(ming) (pool) (suit)
sweep
swing
sweet
sweater

/sl/

slow
sled
slide
sleep(ing)
slip
slipper

/ks/

box
fix
six
rocks

/str/

straw
stripes
street
strong
stranger
strawberries

/skr/

square
squirrel

/μ/ Blends

/br/

broom
brown
break
broke(n)
brush
brother

/dr/

dry
dreamy
drum
drop
drink
dress

/tr/

tree
train
trike
truck
tractor

/gr/

grow
grapes
green
grass
grandma

/kr/

cry(ing)
crawl
cross
cream (ice)
Christmas
crayon

/fr/

frog
friend
fries (french)
freezer
Friday

Appendix B

SOME COMMERCIALLY AVAILABLE COMMUNICATION DEVICES

JANE Y. MURDOCK

Company	*Device(s)*
Communication Skill Builders 3130 N. Dodge Blvd. P. O. Box 42050-F Tucson, AZ 85733	Vocaid
HC Electronics, Inc. 250 Camino Alto Mill Valley, CA 94941	HandiVoice 110 HandiVoice 120
Lars Lindberg Box 3059 S-16103 Bromma, Sweden	Sesam Elektronic AB
POSSUM-Controls Limited East Coast Division P. O. Box 451 Midwood Station Brooklyn, NY 11230	POSSOM Communicator
Prentke Romich Co. 8769 Township Road 515 Shreve, OH 44676-9421	Express I, II, III Vocaid VIP Communicator Memowriter (Sharp) Message Selector MS-2 Autocom

Special thanks to Diane Bristow, M.A., CCC-Sp, Speech/Language Pathologist at Children's Hospital, New Orleans, LA. This list is not comprehensive, but is intended to serve only as a starting point for readers who are not acquainted with computer generated communication devices.

Company	*Device(s)*
	Canon Communicator Superphone Message Selector MS-3 MINSPEAK
Sci-Tronics, Inc. 114 Stillwood Drive Coraopolis, PA 15108	Form-A-Phrase System
SiDiKi Parts Dept. 24 Wilson Avenue NE St. Cloud, NM 56301	SiDiKi System E-Tran
Medelec Limited Manor Way Olk Woking Surrey GU 229JU England	SPLINK
Zygo Industries, INC. P. O. Box 1008 Portland, OR 97207	Memowriter (Sharp) 2-Light Choice Indicator Model 20 Eye Transfer Communication System Models 10, 11, 12 Model 16 Model 16C Model 100 Model 2016 Display Printer (Used with Model 100)

Appendix C

RESOURCE GUIDE FOR COMPUTER TECHNOLOGY FOR THE HANDICAPPED

JANE Y. MURDOCK

THE following information has been adapted from "Technology and Special Education: A Resource Guide" (Bailey & Raimondi, 1984) and "Computer Techology for the Handicapped: A Literature Profile" (Browning and Nave, 1983).

PERIODICALS

Catalyst (Western Center for Microcomputers in Special Education, 1259 El Camino Real, Suite 275, Menlo Park, CA 94025). Intended to interpret, clarify, and communicate microcomputer research and application to special education. Also covers products and current developments.

Closing the Gap (P.O. Box 68, Henderson, MN 56044). Includes information related to special computer modifications and applications with mentally retarded and severely physically handicapped, as well as other handicapped populations.

Communication Outlook (Artificial Language Laboratory, Computer Science Department, Michigan State University, East Lansing, MI 48824). Published by the International Society for Augmentation and Alternative Communication and the Artificial Language Laboratory and Trace Research and Development Center at the University of Wisconsin.

COPH Bulletin (Committee on Personal Computers and the Handicapped, 2030 Irving Park Road, Chicago, IL 60618). Official publication of the Committee on Personal Computers and the Handicapped, a self-help organization intended to enable disabled individuals to use the same computer technologies as the public at large. Its purpose is to search out, evaluate, and share personal computer information deemed relevant to people with disabilities.

The Computing Teacher (1787 Agate Street, University of Oregon, Eugene, OR 97403). Published by the International Council for Computers in Education (ICCE). Good for those who are interested in teaching others about computers. Emphasis is on teaching, computer applications, teacher education, and impact of computers on curriculum.

Journal of Special Education Technology (Exceptional Child Center, Utah State University, UMC 68, Logan, UT 84322). Primarily for researchers, administrators, and teachers. Publishes research, reviews of technology, reports on innovative applications of technology with exceptional children, and general information.

School Microcomputing Bulletin (Learning Publications, Inc., P.O. Box 1326, Holmes Beach, FL 33509). Reports on trends and applications, as well as providing information on sources of materials, software evaluations, workshops, and special field reports by educators.

Teaching, Learning, Computing (Seldin Publishing, Inc., 1061 South Melrose, Suite C., Placentia, CA 92670-7180). Geared toward teachers interested in personal computing. Provides up-to-date reports on computer legislation, special education, administrative planning, and academic disciplines. Includes in-depth product reviews, trends and predictions, management techniques, software test results and evaluations, and profiles of innovative educators.

BOOKS

Computers for the handicapped in special education and rehabilitation: A resource guide (Eugene: University of Oregon, Rehabilitation and Training Center, 1982). Includes over 180 annotated citations from 39 journals, over half dated since 1980. Emphasis is on both computer-assisted and computer-managed instruction in educational and clinical settings.

Dominguez, J., & Waldstein, A. (Eds.), *Educational applications of electronic technology* (Monmouth, OR: WESTAR, 1982). Collection of articles designed to enhance awareness of developments, issues, and applications of electronic technology in education.

Goldenberg, E. P. *Special technology for special children: Computers to serve communication and autonomy in the education of handicapped children* (Baltimore, MD: University Park Press, 1979). Innovative view of computers in special education, including use of LOGO with cerebral palsied, deaf, and autistic students.

Hagen, D. *Microcomputer resource book for special education* (Reston, VA: Reston Publishing Co., 1982). Available through the Council for Exceptional Children. Provides an understanding of the microcomputer as a life competency tool. Shows how computers work for children at home and school. Describes the full spectrum of software and adaptive devices. Looks at disabilities, one at a time, and the computer needs of disability groups. Appendices provide information on over 200 software publishers. Products are organized according to type of disability.

Personal computers and the disabled: A resource guide (Cupertino, CA: Apple Computer, Inc., 1983). Document was prepared as a public service to stimulate research into computer applications for the disabled. Features articles on how computers help the disabled overcome obstacles and limitaitons. Over 60 resources, products for special needs, and organizations are included.

Taber, F. M. *Microcomputers in special education: Selection and decision-making process* (Reston, VA: The Council for Exceptional Children, 1983). Provides an introduction to the microcmputer and its uses in both general and special education. Covers subjects ranging from software considerations to media selection, to elementary programming.

ORGANIZATIONS

Association for the Development of Computer-Based Instructional Systems (ADCIS) (ADCIS Headquarters, Miller Hall 409, Western Washington University, Bellingham, VA 98225). Facilitates communication between product users and developers in an attempt to reduce repetitive efforts. Provides a variety of services, including conferences and workshops, and also sponsors special interest groups, including Educators of the Handicapped.

Association for Special Education Technology (ASET) (P.O. Box 152, Allen, TX 75002). A national affiliate of the Association of Educational Communication and Technology. Established (1) to bring together disciplines sharing a common interest in improving the use of technology in special education, (2) to identify and publicize unique instructional needs of special education students, and (3) to promote improved federal legislation for technology in special education. Publishes *The Journal of Special Education Technology.* Provides an ongoing forum for members to focus on needs of handicapped students who can be assisted through improved technology.

Computer-Using Educators (CUE) (P.O. Box 18547, San Jose, CA 95158). Organization committed to expanding the use of computer technology in education.

The Illinois Council, Congress of Organizations of the Physically Handicapped, Committee on Personal Computers and the Handicapped (COPH-2) (2030 Irving Park Road, Chicago, IL 60618). Seeks out, evaluates, and shares information on hardware, software, software modifications, educational materials developed for disabled people, and uses of computers as part of the personal development of handicapped children. Provides for testing, manufacture, and distribution of low-cost, computer-related hardware. Publishes *Link and Go.*

Michigan Association for Computer Users in Learning (MACUL). (P.O. Box 628,

Westland, MI 48185). Organization of Michigan educators. Coordinates instructional computing activities throughout the state. Sponsors a yearly conference. Membership includes a subscription to the MACUL newsletter. Has some programs for the Apple II, the PET, and the Atari 800.

Technology and Media (TAM) (Dr. Charles McArthur, Membership Chairperson, University of Maryland, Institute of Exceptional Children and Youth, College Park, MD 20742). International association of special education professionals interested in technology and media. Recently organized by members of The Council for Exceptional Children. Formal application has been made to become a division of CEC. TAM is an organization concerned with the impact of technology and media on the diagnosis, treatment, and educational rehabilitation of exceptional persons. Developed and disseminates a journal and newsletter which contain information related to technology and media in special education.

The Young People's LOGO Association (YPLA) (1208 Hillsdale Drive, Richardson, TX 75081). Computer club run for and by young people. *Turtle News* is included with membership, along with access to a software exchange for all popular personal computers which includes teacher- and user-developed software ranging from simple to complex games and educational and business software and software developed by and for the handicapped. Also has an electronic bulletin board and a resource library.

RESOURCE GROUPS

Artifical Language Laboratory (Michigan State University, Computer Science Department, East Lansing, MI 48824). Involved in basic research in the field of computer processing and formal linguistic structure. Research includes speech analysis and synthesis, interspecific communication, pattern recognition of human electromyographic (EMG) signals, and neurolinguistics. Laboratory is also involved in developing vocational and educational aids for the blind.

Center for Computer Assistance to the Disabled (P.O. Box 314, Hurst, TX 76053). Provides a location where disabled persons can gain assistance with the application of microcomputers. Encourages the use of off-the-shelf hardware, currently available technology, and products to aid the education and training of mentally and physically handicapped persons.

MicroSIFT (Northwest Regional Educational Laboratory, 300 S.W. Sixth Avenue, Portland, OR 97204). A clearinghouse for descriptive and evaluative information about microcmputer instructional software and teacher information which is distributed to state and local education agencies and selected commercial and professional periodicals.

Minnesota Educational Computer Consortium (MECC). (3490 Lexington Ave.,

North, Saint Paul, MN 55112). Publisher of training materials and educational courseware for most popular personal computers. Can help any teacher or parent interested in putting personal computers in the classroom. Also has directed a project to develop computer learning packages for use in science, mathematics, and social studies courses. *Network* is an instructional newsletter listing available materials. There is also a catalog available upon request.

National Center for Research in Vocational Education (1960) Kenny Road, Columbus, OH 43210). Provides materials on various aspects of career and vocational education, including programs for special needs populations. Also available are several publications including a discussion guide on microcomputers in vocational education, an administrator's guide to microcomputer resources, and a system for evaluating microcomputer courseware for vocational and technical educators.

SOFTSWAP/CUE. (Microcomputer Center, SMERC Library, San Mateo County Office of Education, 333 Main Street, Redwood City, CA 94063). A joint project of San Mateo County Office of Education and Computer-Using Educators (CUE). Serves as a clearinghouse of public domain educational software. Programs are available free of charge to educators who copy them onto their own disks at the Microcomputer Center or may be ordered for $10. Is also a software exchange. Any educator who contributes an original program on a disk may request any SOFTSWAP disk in exchange. BLOCKS, the courseware development system developed at the California School for the DEAF, and other couseware are available.

Technical Education Research Center, Inc. (TERC) (Computer Resource Center, 8 Eliot Street, Cambridge, MA 02138). Mission is to study social and technological changes and to apply that knowledge to improving education. Currently has two centers: the Special Needs Center and the Technology Center. Publishes a newsletter entitled *Hands On.*

Trace Research and Development Center (314 Waisman Center, University of Wisconsin-Madison, 1500 Highland Avenue, Madison, WI 53705). Studies and develops techniques and aids to augment communication skills of clinical patients in cooperation with the Communications Aids and Systems Clinic of the University of Wisconsin Hospitals. Collects, documents, and disseminates information on these and other communication aids and techniques.

Market Linkage Project for Special Education (LINC Resources, Inc., 3857 North High Street, Suite 225, Columbus, OH 43214). This project though its contact with the Office of Special Education (OSE) of the U.S. Department of Education offers product developers assistance in understanding how to develop educational products to meet national distrubtion standards and to assure that these products are available in classrooms. LINC will provide free technical assistance, help in developing products and assistance in locating a publisher to any project funded by ED/OSE.

Microcomputers in the Schools – Applications in Special Education (SRA Corporation, 901 South Highland Street, Arlington, VA 22004). Will analyze the experiences of local schools currently using microcomputers with programs for the handicapped and then develop and disseminate research-based information to assist introducing microcomputers in special education programs.

NETWORKS

Project C.A.I.S.H. (Computer-Assisted Instruction and Support for the Handicapped) (3450 Gozio Road, Sarasota, FL 33580). A Title VI-B project funded through the state of Florida. Provides hardware and software for all exceptionalities, teacher training, and implementation workshops. First year of project was devoted to physically handicapped; second year to the mentally and emotionally handicapped. Presently addressing remaining exceptionalities.

project EduTech (JWK International Corp. 7617 Little River Turnpike, Annandale, VA 22003). Provides technical assistance to state and local education agencies in use of technology in special education. Selects widespread special education issues on which to focus each year. Develops reports and otherwise disseminates information on technological advances that may resolve these issues. Maintains information system on technological advances.

Project RECIPE (Research Exchange for Computerized Individualized Programs of Education) (1001) South School Avenue, Sarasota, FL 33577). A nationally validated instructional management system designed to help educators create and implement individualized education programs (IEP's). System includes instructional objectives, criterion-referenced assessment system, and instructional strategies. Has a management component designed to track and record student progress. Provides progress reports. May be used at classroom, building, or district level.

SECTOR Project (Exceptional Child Center, UMC-68, Utah State University, Logan, UT 84322). State-funded special education computer technology resource located at Utah State University. Conducts overviews of adaptive and communication devices. Reviews courseware for handicapped students and software for special education management. Maintains bibliographic information base for special education. Also conducts research on the intractive videodisc.

CLEARINGHOUSES

Apple Computer Clearinghouse for the Handicapped (Prentke Romich Company, RD 2, Bos 191, Serene, OH 44676). Clearinghouse for software.

Computer Assisted Instruction for Handicapped Children and Youth and *Use of Computers in Regular and Special Education Teacher Education* (CEC Publication Sales, 1920 Association Drive, Reston, VA 22091). Clearinghouse for literature available through CEC/ERIC Computer Search Reprints.

Trace Software Registry and Listing of Programs Adapted for Rehabilitaiton Applications with Microcomputers (Trace Research and Development Center for Severely communicatively Handicapped, University of Wisconsin, Madison, WI 53705). Clearinghouse for software.

REFERENCES

Alberto, P., Jobes, N., Sizemore, A., & Doran, D. (1980). A comparison of individual and group instruction across response tasks. *The Journal of the Association for the Severely Handicapped, 5,* 285-293.

Alberto, P. A., & Troutman, A. C. (1982). *Applied behavior analysis for teachers: Influencing student performance.* Columbus, OH: Charles E. Merrill.

Allen, G. J. (1973). Case study: Implementation of behavior modification techniques in summer camp settings. *Behavior Therapy, 4,* 570-575.

Anthony, D. (1971). *Seeing essential English.* Anaheim, CA: Educational Services Division, Anaheim School District.

Axelrod, S. (1983). *Behavior modification for the classroom teacher* (2nd ed.). New York: McGraw-Hill.

Ayllon, T., Layman, D., & Kandel, H. J. (1975). A behavioral-educational alternative to drug control of hyperactive children. *Journal of Applied Behavior Analysis, 8,* 137-146.

Baer, D. M., Peterson, R. F., & Sherman, J. A. (1967). The development of imitation by reinforcing behavioral similarity to a model. *Journal of Experimental Analysis of Behavior, 10,* 405-416.

Baer, D. M., Wolf, M. M., & Risley, T. R. (1968). Some current dimensions of applied behavior analysis. *Journal of Applied Behavior Analysis, 1,* 91-97.

Bailey, M. N., & Raimondi, S. L. (1984). Technology and special education: A resource guide. *Teaching Exceptional Children, 16,* 273-277.

Bandura, A. (1969). *Principles of behavior modification.* New York: Holt, Rinehart, & Winston.

Bandura, A. (Ed.). (1971). *Psychological modeling: Conflicting theories.* New York: Aldine/Atherton.

Barlow, D. H., & Hayes, S. D. (1979). Alternating treatments design: One strategy for comparing the effects of two treatments in a single subject. *Journal of Applied Behavior Analysis, 12,* 199-210.

Barrera, R. D., & Sulzer-Azaroff, B. (1983). An alternating treatment comparison of oral and total communication training program with echolalic autistic children. *Journal of Applied Behavior Analysis, 16,* 379-394.

Bates, E. (1976). *Language and context.* New York: Academic Press.

Bates, E. (1979). *The emergence of symbols: Cognition and communication in infancy.* New York: Academic Press.

Bayley, N. (1969). *Bayley scales of infant development.* New York: The Psychological Corp.

Becker, W. C., Engelmann, S., & Thomas, D. R. (1971). *Teaching: A course in applied psychology.* Chicago: Science Research Associates.

Bell, S., & Cady, P. (1984, March). *The use of computers to manage instruction in special education re-*

source rooms. Paper presented at the meeting of the 1984 International Conference of the Association for Children and Adults with Learning Disabilities, New Orleans, LA.

Bennett, R. E. (1982). Applications of microcomputer technology to special education. *Exceptional Children, 49,* 106-113.

Berko, J. (1958). The child's learning of English morphology. *Word, 14,* 359-375.

Bijou, S. W., & Baer, D. M. (1967). *Child development: Readings in experimental analysis.* New York: Appleton-Century-Crofts.

Bliss, C. K., (1965). *Semantography-Blissymbolics.* Sydney, Australia: Semantography Publications. (Distributed by C. K. Bliss, P. O. Box 222, Coogee 2034, Sydney, Astralia.)

Bornstein, H. (1973). A description of some current sign systems designed to represent English. *American Annals of the Deaf, 118,* 454-463.

Bornstein, H. (1974). Signed English, a manual approach. *Journal of Speech and Hearing Disorders, 39,* 330-343.

Bricker, W. A., & Bricker, D. D. (1974). An early language training strategy. In R. L. Schiefelbusch & L. L. Lloyd (Eds.), *Language perspectives — Acquisition, retardation, and intervention* (pp. 431-468). Baltimore: University Park Press.

Bristow, D. (1983, October). *Communication aids.* Paper presented at a meeting on nonspeech communication/electronic aids by the Department of Speech, Language & Audiology of Children's Hospital, New Orleans, LA.

Brookshire, R. H. (1967). Speech pathology and the experimental analysis of behavior. *Journal of Speech and Hearing Disorders, 32,* 215-227.

Brown, N. P. (1982). CAMEO: Computer-assisted management of educational objectives. *Exceptional Children, 49,* 151-153.

Brown, R., & Bellugi, U. (1964). Three processes in the child's acquisition of syntax. In E. Lenneberg (Ed.), *New directions in the study of language* (pp. 131-161). Cambridge: MIT Press.

Browning, P., & Nave, G. (1983). Computer technology for the handicapped: A literature profile. *The Computing Teacher, 10,* 56-59.

Bruner, J. S. (1975). The ontogenesis of speech acts. *Journal of Child Language, 2,* 1-19.

Budoff, M., & Hutten L. R. (1982). Microcomputers in special education: Promises and pitfalls. *Exceptional Children, 49,* 123-128.

Bzoch, K. R., & League, R. (1971). *Assessing language skills in infancy: A handbook for the multidimensional analysis of emergent language.* Baltimore: University Park Press.

Cain, E. J. (1984a, March). *Microcomputers — A technology for all; a normalization agent for many — Daily living and functional skill proficiencies for the learning disabled.* Paper presented at the meeting of the 1984 International Conference of the Association for Children and Adults with Learning Disabilities, New Orleans, LA.

Cain, E. J. (1984b). The challenge of technology: Educating the exceptional child for the world of tomorrow. *Teaching Exceptional Children, 16,* 239-241.

Carr, E. G. (1979). Teaching autistic children to use sign language: Some research issues. *Journal of Autism and Developmental Disorders, 9,* 345-359.

Carr, E. G. (1980). Generalization of treatment effects following educational intervention with autistic children and youth. In B. Wilcox & A. Thompson (Eds.), *Critical issues in educating autistic children and youth* (pp. 118-134). Washington, DC: The National Society for Children and Adults with Autism.

Carr, E. G., Binkoff, J. A., Kologinsky, E., & Eddy, M. (1978). Acquisition of sign language by autistic children I: Expressive labeling. *Journal of Applied Behavior Analysis, 11,* 489-501.

Carr, E. G., & Kologinsky, E. (1983). Acquisition of sign language by autistic children II: Spontaneity and generalization effects. *Journal of Applied Behavior Analysis, 16,* 297-314.

Carrier, J. K., Jr. (1974). Nonspeech noun usage training with severely and profoundly retarded children. *Journal of Speech and Hearing Research, 17,* 510-517.

Carrier, J. K., Jr. (1976). Application of a nonspeech language system with the severely language handicapped. In L. L. Lloyd (Ed.), *Communication assessment and intervention strategies* (pp. 523-547). Baltimore: University Park Press.

Carrier, J. K., Jr., & Peak, T. (1975). *Non-speech language imitation program.* Lawrence, KS: H & H Enterprises.

Cassidy-Bronson, S., Miller, E., & Slaughter, J. C. (1984, March). *Microcomputer management of special education.* Paper presented at the meeting of the 1984 International Conference of the Association for Children and Adults with Learning Disabilities, New Orleans, LA.

Cavallaro, C. C. (1983). Language interventions in natural settings. *Teaching Exceptional Children,* 65-70.

Clark, C. R., Davies, C. O., & Woodcock, R. W. (1974). *Standard rebus glossary.* Circle Pines, MN: American Guidance Service.

Clark, C., Moores, D., & Woodcock, R. (1975a). *The Minnesota early langage development sequence: Teacher's manual. Development kit #1.* Minneapolis: University of Minnesota Research, Development and Demonstration Center in Education of Handicapped Children.

Clark, C., Moores, D., & Woodcock, R. (1975b). *The Minnesota early language development sequence: Parent's manual. Development kit #2.* Minneapolis: University of Minnesota Research, Development and Demonstration Center in Education of Handicapped Children.

Colby, K. M. (1973). The rationale for computer-based treatment of language difficulties in nonspeaking autistic children. *Journal of Autism and Childhood Schizophrenia, 3,* 254-260.

Cole, M. L., & Cole, J. T. (1981). *Effective intervention with the language impaired child.* Rockville, MD: Aspen.

Dale, P. S. (1972). *Language development: Structure and function.* New York: Holt, Rinehart and Winston.

Damasco, P., & Foulds, R. (1982). A new horizon for non-vocal communication devices. *Byte, 7,* 166-182.

Daniloff, J. K., & Shafer, A. (1981). A gestural communication program for severely and profoundly handicapped children. *Language, Speech, and Hearing Services in Schools, 12,* 258-267.

Dever, R. B. (1974). Discussion summary — Nonspeech communication. In R. L. Schiefelbusch & L. L. Lloyd (Eds.), *Language perspectives — Acquisition, retardation, and intervention* (pp. 419-427). Baltimore: University Park Press.

Doke, L. A., & Risley, T. R. (1972). The organization of day-care environments: Required vs. optional activities. *Journal of Applied Behavior Analysis, 5,* 405-420.

Duker, P. C., & Morsink, H. (1984). Acquisition and cross-setting generalization of manual signs with severely retarded individuals. *Journal of Applied Behavior Analysis, 17,* 93-103.

Engel, D. C., Brandriet, S. E., Erickson, K. M., Gronhovd, K. D., & Gunderson, G. C. (1966). Carryover. *Journal of Speech and Hearing Disorders, 31,* 227-233.

Ervin, S. M. (1964). Imitation and structural change in children's langauge. In E. H. Lenneberg (Ed.), *New directions in the study of language* (pp. 168-189). Cambridge, MA: MIT Press.

Ervin-Tripp, S. (1971). An overview of theories of grammatical development. In D. I. Slobin (Ed.), *The ontogenesis of grammar* (pp. 189-212). New York: Academic Press.

Faw, G. D., Reid, D. H., Schepis, M. J., Fitzgerald, J. R., & Welty, P. A. (1981). Involving institutional staff in the development and maintenance of sign language skills with profoundly retarded persons. *Journal of Applied Behavior Analysis, 14,* 411-423.

Fernald, G. M. (1943). *Remedial techniques in basic school subjects. New York: McGraw-Hill.*

Fitzgerald, E. (1966). Straight language for the deaf. Washington: DC: The Volta Bureau.

Foulds, R. A. (1982). Applications of microcomputersin the education of the physically disabled child. *Exceptional Children, 49,* 155-162.

Fristoe, M. (1975). *Language intervention systems of the retarded.* Decatur, AL: Lurleen B. Wallace Development Center.

Fulwiler, R. L., & Fouts, R. S. (1976). Acquisition of American sign language by a noncommunicating autistic child. *Journal of Autism and Childhood Schizophrenia, 6,* 43-51.

Garcia, E. (1974). The training and generalization of a conversational speech form in nonverbal retardates. *Journal of Applied Behavior Analysis, 7,* 137-149.

Gardner, R., & Gardner, B. (1969). Teaching sign language to a chimpanzee. *Science, 165,* 664-672.

Gray, B. B., & Ryan, B. P. (1973). *A langauge program for the nonlanguage child.* Champaign, IL: Research Press.

Guess, D., Sailor, W., & Baer, D. M. (1974). To teach language to retarded children. In R. L. Schiefelbusch & L. L. Lloyd (Eds.), *Language perspectives — Acquisition, retardation, and intervention* (pp. 529-563). Baltimore: University Park Press.

Guess, D., Sailor, W., & Baer, D. M. (1976). *Functional speech and langauge training for the severely handicapped: Parts I and II.* Lawrence, KS: H & H Enterprises.

Guess, D., Sailor, W., Rutherford, G., & Baer, D. M. (1968). An experimental analysis of linguistic development: The productive use of the plural morpheme. *Journal of Applied Behavior Analysis, 1,* 297-306.

Gustason, G., Pfetzing, D., & Zawolkow, E. (1972). *Signing exact English.* Rossmoor, CA: Modern Signs Press.

Hall, R. V. (1971). Responsive teaching: Focus on measurement and research in the classroom and the home. *Focus on Exceptional Children, 3,* 1-8.

Hall, R. V. (1974). *Managing behavior, part 1: Behavior modification: The measurement of behavior* (Rev. ed.). Lawrence, KS: H & H Enterprises.

Hall, R. V. (1975). *Managing behavior, part 2: Behavior modification: Basic principles* (Rev. ed.). Lawrence, KS: H & H Enterprises.

Hall, R. V., & Fox, R. G. (1977). Changing-criterion designs: An alternate applied behavior analysis procedures. InrB. C. Etzel, J. M. LeBlanc, & D. M. Baer (Eds.), *New developments in behavioral research: Theory, method, and application. In honor of Sydney W. Bijou* (pp. 151-166). Hillsdale, NJ: Lawrence Erlbaum.

Hall, R. V., & Fox, R. G. (1978). *The responsive teaching-parenting model transparency kit: Instructor's manual* (Rev. ed.). Lawrence, KS: H & H Enterprises.

Handleman, J. S. (1979). Generalization by autistic-type children of verbal responses across settings. *Journal of Applied Behavior Analysis, 12,* 273-282.

Hannaford, A., & Sloane, E. (1981). Microcomputers: Powerful learning tools with proper programming. *Teaching Exceptional Children, 14,* 54-57.

Hannaford, A. E. (1983). Microcomputers in special education: Some new opportunities, some old prolems. *The Computing Teacher, 10,* 11-17.

Hannaford, A. E., & Taber, F. M. (1982). Microcomputer software for the handicapped: Development and evaluation. *Exceptional Children, 49,* 137-142.

Harris, D., & Vanderheiden, G. C. (1980). Enhancing the development of communicative interaction. In R. L. Schiefelbusch (Ed.), *Nonspeech language and communication: Analysis and intervention* (Vol. 4) (pp. 227-257). Baltimore: University Park Press.

Hart, B., & Risley, T. R. (1974). Using preschool materials to modify the language of disadvantaged children. *Journal of Applied Behavior Analysis, 7,* 243-256.

Hart, B., & Risley, T. R. (1975) Incidental teaching of langauge in the preschool. *Journal of Applied Behavior Analysis, 8,* 411-420.

Hart, B., & Risley, T. R. (1980). In vivo language intervention: Unanticipated general effects. *Journal of Applied Behavior Analysis, 13,* 407-432.

Hart, B., & Rogers-Warren, A. (1978). A milieu approach to teaching langauge. In R. L.

Schiefelbush (Ed.), *Language intervention strategies: Language intervention series* (Vol. 2) (pp. 193-235). Baltimore: University Park Press.
Hartmann, B. (1975). Ordered list of environmentally useful words. In J. Y. Murdock & B. Hartmann, *A language development program: Imitative gestures to basic syntactic structures* (pp. 25-35). Salt Lake City: Word Making Productions.
Hartmann, D. P., & Hall, R. V. (1976). The changing criterion design. *Journal of Applied Behavior Analysis, 9,* 527-532.
Hasselbring, T., & Hamlett, C. (1983). *AIMSTAR: A data management and decision-making system.* Portland, OR: ASIEP Education Co.
Hasselbring, T., & Hamlett, C. (1984). Planning and managing instruction: Computer-based decision making. *Teaching Exceptional Children, 16,* 248-252.
Hersen, M., & Barlow, D. H. (1976). *Single-case experimental designs: Strategies for studying behavior change.* New York: Pergamon Press.
Higginbotham, D. J., & Yoder, D. E. (1982). Communication within natural conversational interaction: Implications for severe communicatively impaired persons. *Topics in Language Disorders: Communication Interaction Strategies for the Severely, Communicatively Impaired, 2,* 1-19.
Hinerman, P.S. (1983). *Teaching autistic children to communicate.* Rockville, MD: Aspen.
Hodges, P., & Deich, R. F. (1979). Language intervention strategies with manipulable symbols. In R. L. Schiefelbusch & J. H. Hollis (Eds.), *:Language intervention from ape to child* (pp. 419-440). Baltimore: University Park Press.
Hofmeister, A. M. (1982). Microcomputers in perspective. *Exceptional Children, 49,* 115-121.
Holland, J. G., & Skinner, B. F. (1961). *The analysis of behavior.* New York: McGraw-Hill.
Hollis, J. H., & Carrier, J. K., Jr. (1978). Intervention strategies for nonspeech children. In R.L. Schiefelbusch (Ed.), *Language intervention strategies* (pp. 56-100). Baltimore: University Park Press.
Hurlbut, B. I., Iwata, B. A., & Green, J. D. (1982). Nonvocal language acquisition in adolescents with severe physical disabilities: Blissymbol versus iconic stimulus formats. *Journal of Applied Behavior Analysis, 15,* 241-258.
Johnson, D. J., & Myklebust, H. R. (1964). *Learning disabilities: Educational principles and practices.* New York: Grune & Stratton.
Johnston, J. M., & Johnston, G. T. (1972). Modificationof consonant speech-sound articulation in young children. *Journal of Applied Behavior Analysis, 5,* 233-246.
Kamp, S. (1983). *Training manual for microcomputers in special education* (draft). Reston, VA: The Council for Exceptional Children.
Kazdin, A. E., & Bootzin, R. R. (1972). The token economy: An evaluative review. *Journal of Applied Behavior Analysis, 5,* 343-372.
Kent, L. (1974). *Language acquisition program for the severely retarded.* Champaign, IL: Research Press.
Kirschner, A., Algozzine, B., & Abbott, T. B. (1979). Manual communication systems: A comparison and its implications. *Education and Training of the Mentally Retarded, 14,* 5-10.
Koegel, R. L., & Rincover, A. (1974). Treatment of psychotic children in a classroom environment: I. Learning in a large group. *Journal of Applied Behavior Analysis, 7,* 45-59.
Kopchick, G. A., & Lloyd, L. L. (1976). Total communication for the severely language impaired: A 24-hour approach. In L. L. Lloyd (Ed.), *Communication assessment and intervention strategies* (pp. 501-521). Baltimore: University Park Press.
Kopchick, G. A., Rombach, D. W., & Smilovitz, R. (1975). A total communication environment in an institution. *Mental Retardation, 13,* 22-23.
LaVigna, G. W. (1977). Communication training in mute autistic adolescents. *Journal of Autism and Childhood Schizophrenia, 7,* 135-144.
Lloyd, L. L. (Ed.). (1976). *Communication assessment and intervention strategies.* Baltimore: Univer-

sity Park Press.

Lovaas, O. I. (1977). A program for the establishment of speech in psychotic children. In J. K. Wing (Ed.), *Early childhood autism* (pp. 115-144). Oxford: Pergamon.

Lovaas, O. I., Berberich, J. P., Perloff, B. f., & Schaeffer, B. (1966). Acquisition of imitative speech by schizophrenic children. *Science, 151,* 705-707.

Lucas, E. V. (1980). *Semantic and pragmatic language disorders: Assessment and remediation.* Rockville, MD: Aspen.

Luttner, S. (1981). Computers for the handicapped. *Apple Magazine, 2,* 26-29.

MacDonald, J. D. (1982). *Language through conversation.* Columbus, OH: Ohio State University.

MacDonald, J. D., & Horstmeier, D. S. (1978). *Environmental language intervention program.* Columbus, OH: Charles E. Merrill.

MacDonald, J. D., & Nickols, M. (1974). *Environmental language inventory.* Columbus, OH: Charles E. Merrill.

Marshall, N. & Hegrenes, J. (1972). The use of written language as a communication system for an autistic child. *Journal of Speech and Hearing Disordes, 37,* 258-261.

Mayberry, R. (1976). If a chimp can learn sign language, surely my nonverbal client can too. *Asha, 18,* 223-228.

McDonald, E. T. (1980). Early identification and treatment of children at risk for speech development. In R. L. Schiefelbusch (Ed.), *Nonspeech language and communication: Analysis and intervention* (pp. 49-79). Baltimore: University Park Press.

McDonald, E. T., & Schultz, A. R. (1973). Communication boards for cerebral palsied children. *Journal of Speech and Hearing Disorders, 38,* 73-88.

McGee, G. G., Krantz, P. J., Mason, D., & McClannahan, L. E. (1983). A modified incidental-teaching procedure for autistic youth: Acquisition and generalization of receptive labels. *Journal of Applied Behavior Analysis, 16,* 329-338.

McLean, J., & Snyder-McLean, L. K. (1978). *A transactional approach to early language training: Derivationof a model sytem.* Columbus, OH: Charles E. Merrill.

McLean, L. P., & McLean, J. E. (1978). A language training program for nonverbal autistic children. In M. Lahey (Ed.), *Readings in childhood language disorders* (pp. 418-426). New York: John Wiley & Sons.

McNaughton, S., & Kates, B. (1980). The application of Blissymbolics. In R. L. Schiefelbusch (Ed.), *Nonspeech language and communication: Analysis and intervention* (pp. 303-321). Baltimore: University Park Press.

Mehrabian, A. (1972). *Nonverbal communication.* Chicago: Aldine-Atherton Press.

Menyuk, P. (1972). *The development of speech.* New York: Bobbs-Merrill.

Miller, M. L. (1984, March). *Workshops on Logo: Strategies for learning.* Paper presented at the meeting of at the 1984 International Conference of the Association for Children and Adults with Learning Disabilities, New Orleans, LA.

Moores, D. F. (1980). Alternative communication modes. In R.L. Schiefelbusch (Ed.), *Nonspeech language and communication: Analysis and intervention* (pp. 27-47). Baltimore: University Park Press.

Mulac, A., & Tomlinson, C. N. (1977). Generalization of an operant remediation program for syntax with language delayed children. *Journal of Communication Disorders, 10,* 231-243.

Murdock, J. Y. (1978a). Behavior modification. In F. W. Litton, *Educationof the trainable-mentally retarded: Curriculum, methods, materials* (pp. 65-91). St. Louis: C. V. Mosby.

Murdock, J. Y. (1978b). A non-oral expressive communication program designed for a nonverbal retardate. *Journal of Childhood Communication Disorders, 2,* 18-25.

Murdock, J. Y., Garcia, E., & Hardman, M. L. (1977). Generalizing articulation training with trainable mentally retarded subjects. *Journal of Applied Behavior analysis, 10,* 717-734.

Murdock, J. Y., & Hartmann, B. (1975). *A language development program: Imitative gestures to basic syntactic structures.* Salt Lake City: Word Making Productions.

Murdock, J. Y., & Sabrio, L. D. (1983). Effects of presentation rate and consequences on immediate and long-term recall of learning disabled students: A combination multiple baseline, time-series analysis of single-subject data. In W. M. Cruickshank & E. Tash, *Academics and beyond: The best of ACLD* (Vol. 4) (pp. 27-49). Syracuse, NY: Syracuse University Press.

Myers, P. I., & Hammill, D. D. (1976). *Methods for learning disorders* (2nd ed.). New York: John Wiley and Sons.

Nave, G., Browning, P., & Carter, J. (1983). *Computer technology for the handicapped in special education and rehabilitation: A resource guide.* Eugene, OR: International Council for Computers in Education, University of Oregon.

Nietupski, J., Scheutz, G., & Ockwood, L. (1980). The delivery of communication therapy services to severely handicapped students: A plan for change. *Journal of the Association for the Severely handicapped, 5,* 13-23.

O'Brien, F. Azrin, N. H., & Henson, K. (1969). Increased communication of chronic mental patients by reinforcement and by response priming. *Journal of Applied Behavior analysis, 2,* 23-29.

Panyon, M. C. (1975). *Managing behavior, part 4: New ways to teach new skills* (Rev. ed.). Lawrence, KS: H & H Enterprises.

Premack, A. J., & Premack, D. (1972). Teaching language to an ape. *Scientific American, 227,* 92-99.

Premack, D. (1959). Toward empirical behavior laws: Positive reinforcement. *Psychological Review, 66,* 219-233.

Premack, D. (1970). A functional analysis of language. *Journal of Experimental Analysis of Behavior, 14,* 107, 125.

Premack, D. (1971). Language in chimpanzees? *Science, 172,* 808-822.

Premack, D., & Premack, A. (1974). Teaching visual language to apes and language-deficient persons. in R. L. Schiefelbusch & L. L. Lloyd (Eds.), *Language perspectives — Acquisition, retardation, and intervention* (pp. 347-376). Baltimore: University Park Press.

Redd, W. H., & Birnbrauer, J. S. (1969). Adults as discriminative stimuli for different reinforcement contingencies with retarded children. *Journal of Experimental Child Psychology, 7,* 440-447.

Rees, N. S. (1975). Imitation and language development. *Journal of Speech and Hearing Disorders, 40,* 339-350.

Remington, B., & Clark S. (1983). Acquisition of expressive signing by autistic children: An avaluation of the relative effects of simultaneous communication and sign-alone training. *Journal of Applied Behavior Analysis, 16,* 315-327.

Risley, T. R.,& Wolf, M. M. (1967). Establishment of functional speech in echolalic children. *Behavior Research and therapy, 5,* 73-88.

Roane, G. (1983, October). *Amer-Ind.* Paper presented at a meeting on nonspeech communication/electronic aids by the Department of Speech, Language & Audiology of Children's Hospital, New Orleans, LA.

Roe, F. H. (1948). Their right to learn. *Hygeia, 26,* 348-394.

Rogers-Warren, A., & Warren, S. F. (1980). Mands for verbalization: Facilitating the display of newly trained language in children. *Behavior Modification, 4,* 361-382.

Sanders, E. K. (1972). When are speech sounds learned? *Journal of Speech and Hearing Disorders, 37,* 55-63.

Sayre, J. M. (1963). Communication for the nonverbal cerebral palsied. *C. P. Review, 24.* 6.

Schaeffer, B. (1978). Teaching spontaneous sign language to nonverbal children: Theory and method. *Sign Language Studies, 21,* 317-352.

Schaeffer, B. (1980). Spontaneous language through signed speech. In R. L. Schiefelbusch (Ed.). *Nonspeech language and communication: Analysis and intervention* (pp. 421-446). Baltimore: University Park Press.

Schaeffer, B., Musil, A., & Kollinzas, G. (1980). *Total communication: A signed speech program for nonverbal children.* Champaign, IL: Research Press.

Schiefelbusch, R. L. (1974). Summary. In R. L. Schiefelbusch & L. L. Lloyd, *Language perspectives — Acquisition, retardation, and intervention* (pp. 647-660). Baltimore: University Park Press.

Schiefelbusch, R. L. (Ed.). (1980). *Nonspeech language and communication Analysis and intervention.* Baltimore: University Park Press.

Schiefelbusch, R. L., & Hollis, J. H. (Eds.(. (1979). *Language intervention from ape to child.* Baltimore: University Park Press.

Schiefelbusch, r L., & Hollis, J. H. (1980). A general system for nonspeech language. In R. L. Schiefelbusch (Ed.), *Nonspeech language and communication: Analysis and intervention* (pp. 5-23). Baltimore: University Park Press.

Schiefelbusch, R. L., & Lloyd, L. L. (1974). *Language perspectives — Acquisition, retardation, and intervention.* Baltimore: University Park Press.

Schiffman, G., Tobin, D., & Cassidy-Bronson, S. (1982). Personal computers for the learning disabled. *Journal of Learning Disabilities, 15,* 422-425.

Schuler, A. L. (1980). Teaching functional language. In B. Wilcox & A. Thompson (Eds.), *Critical issues in educating autistic children and youth* (pp. 154-178), Washington, DC: The National Society for Children and Adults with Autism.

Schuler, A. L., & Baldwin, M. (1981). Nonspeech communication and childhood autism. *Language, Speech, and Hearing Services in Schools, 12,* 246-257.

Shane, H. C. (1980). Approaches to assessing the communication of non-oral persons. In R. L. Schiefelbusch (Ed.), *Nonspeech language and communication: Analysis and intervention* (pp. 197-224). Baltimore: University Park Press.

Sherman, J. A. (1971). Imitation and language development. In H. W. Reese (Ed.), *Advances in child development and behavior* (Vol. 6) (pp. 239-272). New York: Academic Press.

Sidman, M. (1960). *Tactics of scientific research.* New York: Basic Books.

Silverman, F. L. (1980). *Communication for the Speechless.* Englewood Cliffs, NJ: Prentice-Hall.

Silverman, H., McNaughton, S., & Kates, B. (1978). *Handbook of Blissymbolics.* Canada: Blissymbolics Communication Institute.

Skelley, M. (1979). *Amer-ind gestural code based on universal American Indian hand talk.* New York: Elsevier North Holland.

Skelley, M. Schinsky, L., Smith, R., Donaldson, R., & Griffin, J. (1975). American Indian sign: A gestural communicatio system for the speechless. *Archives of Physical Medicine and Rehabilitation, 56,* 156-160.

Skelley, M., Schinsky, L., Smith, R. W., & Fust, R. S. (1974). American Indian sign (Amerind) as a facilitator of verbalization in the oral apraxic. *Journal of Speech and Hearing Disorders, 39,* 445-456.

Skinner, B. F. (1957). *Verbal behavior.* New York: Appleton-Century-Crofts.

Sloane, H. N., Buckholdt, D. R., Jenson, W. R., & Crandall, J. A. (1979). *Structured teaching: A design for classroom management & instruction.* Champaign, IL: Research Press.

Sloane, H. N., Jr., Johnston, M. K., & Harris, F. R. (1968). In H. N. Sloene, Jr. & B. D. MacAulay (Eds.), *Operant procedures in remedial speech ang language trainng* (pp. 77-101). Boston: Houghton Mifflin.

Sloane, H. N., Jr., & MacAulay, B. D. (Eds.). (1968). *Operant procedures in remedial speech and language training.* Boston: Houghton Mifflin.

Slobin, D. I. (1967). Imitation and grammatical development in children. In N. S. Endler, L. R. Boulter, & H. Osser (Eds.), *Contemporary issues in developmental psychology* (pp. 437-443).

New York: Holt, Rinehart and Winston.

Spring, C. (1984, March). *Computer applications in reading instruction.* Paper presented at the meeting of the 1984 International Conference of the Association for Children and Adults with Learning Disabilities, New Orleans, LA.

Sternberg, L., Battle, C., & Hill, J. (1980). Prelanguage communication programming for the severely and profoundly handicapped. *Journal of the Associaiton for the Severely Handicapped, 5,* 224-233.

Stokes, T. F., & Baer, D. M. (1977). An implicit technology of generalization. *Journal of Applied Behavior analysis, 10,* 349-367.

Stokes, T. F., Baer, D. M., & Jackson, R. L. (1974). Programming the generalization of a greeting response in four retarded children. *Journal of Applied Behavior Analysis, 7,* 599-610.

Striefel, S. (1974). *Managing behavior, part 7: Teaching a child to imitate.* Lawrence, KS: H & H Enterprises.

Taber, F. M. (1983). *Microcomputer in special education: Selection and decision making process.* Reston, VA: The Council for Exceptional Children.

Tawney, J. W., & Gast, D. L. (1984). *Single subject research in special education.* Columbus, OH: Charles E. Merrill.

Trachtman, P. (1984). Putting computers into the hands of children without language. *Smithsonian, 14,* 42-51.

Trantham, C. R., & Pedersen, J. K. (1976). *Normal language development: The key to diagnosis and therapy for language-disordered children.* Baltimore: The Williams & Wilkins Co.

Uzgiris, I. C., & Hunt, J. M. (1975). *Assessment in early infancy.* Urbana: IL: University of Illinois Press.

Vanderheiden, G. (1981). Practical applications of microcomputers to aid the handicapped. *Computer, 14,* 54-61.

Vanderheiden, G. (1982). *Blissapple Manual.* Madison, WI: Trace Center, University of Wisconsin.

Vanderheiden, G. C. (Ed.) (1978). *Non-vocal communication resource book.* Baltimore: University Park Press.

Vanderheiden, G., & Grilley, K. (Eds.). (1976). *Non-vocal communication techniques and aids for the severely physically handicapped.* Baltimore: University Park Press.

Vanderheiden, G., & Harris-Vanderheiden, D. (1976). Communication techniques and aids for non-vocal severely handicapped. In L. L. Lloyd (Ed.), *Communication assessment and intervention strategies* (pp. 607-652). Baltimore: University Park Press.

Wacker, D. (September, 1983). *Microswitches.* Paper presented at the Meeting of Special School District #1, Department of Education, State of Louisiana, Baton Rouge, LA.

Wampler, D. (1971). *Linguistics of visual English.* Santa Rosa, CA: Santa Rosa Public Schools.

Wertz, F. C., Wertz, J. E., & Kehrberg, K. T. (1983). *Blissboard.* St. Paul, MN: Minnesota Educational Computing Consortium.

Woodcock, R. W., Clark, C. R., & Davies, C. O. (1968). *Peabody rebus reading program.* Circle Pines, MN: American Guidance Service.

Woolman, D. H. (1980). A presymbolic training program. In R. L. Schiefelbusch (Ed.), *Nonspeech language and communication: Analysis and intervention* (pp. 325-347). Baltimore: University Park Press.

AUTHOR INDEX

AUTHOR INDEX